OWN YOUR HEALTH

SWIPE RIGHT FOR BETTER HEALTH

DR. VIKRAM VENKATESWARAN

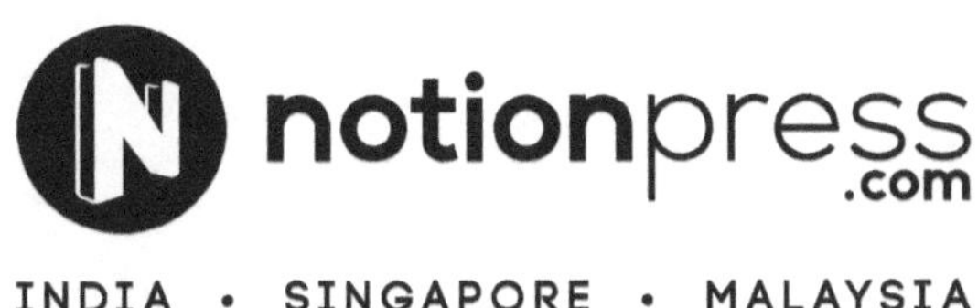

Notion Press

No.8, 3rd Cross Street
CIT Colony, Mylapore
Chennai, Tamil Nadu – 600004

First Published by Notion Press 2021
Copyright © Vikram Venkateswaran 2021
All Rights Reserved.

ISBN 978-1-63745-400-8

Contents

SECTION 3: HEALTHCARE INITIATIVES BY THE GOVERNMENT

Acknowledgements

This book is a result of 43 years spent in healthcare. Growing up in a family that took its health seriously can be the best initiation for someone to take up a career in healthcare. For that I want to thank my parents, the late Dr. Prathima Venkateswaran, a healthcare pioneer and my mother, and my father R. Venkateswaran for trying so many things in his life to maintain his health, To my grandparents, specially my Grandmother, the late Mrs. Rukmani Ramanan for giving me so much confidence as a child and reminding me the moral of the story of the Hare and Tortoise-incidentally tortoises live longer and healthier lives…

I want to thank all my teachers and professors-from DPS RK Puram, MCODS Manipal and IMT Ghaziabad for helping me on this journey. Manipal has been a strong influence in my life-always thinking forward, bringing in innovation, and new approaches to care has been a guiding light for me for many years.

I want to thank all the doctors that have kept me healthy all these years: Dr. Jain, Dr. Anil Kunwar, Dr. P K Gupta, Dr. Usha Rajamany, Dr. Oliver Rodriguez to name a few.

I want to thank the organizations that I worked for that gave me access to major healthcare systems globally and helped me understand what we can learn from these systems.

I want to thank Archana Venkat, my biggest critic for editing the book and being very strict about the kind of content that went into it and Dr. Sumeet Kad for reviewing the healthcare content and checking for factual correctness.

The healthcare industry has given me the opportunity to work with some of the brightest and sharpest minds in the country. I want to thank Ravi Ramaswamy for being a mentor and a coach. He is one of my biggest inspirations to write this book and his agreeing to write the foreword is a big honor for me. Dr. Sudhakar Varanasi is another giant in the healthcare space, being the pioneer of 108 ambulance service. He has inspired me with a simple phone call and I am forever indebted to him for having faith in my abilities.

I want to thank Rajesh Batra, a senior from IMT Ghaziabad and fellow Dilliwala, for his guidance and continued encouragement.

Many people were involved in the creation of this book, some provided content and others reviewed it, Dr. Abhyan Kumar, classmate and good friend for contributing the section on taking care of the eyes, Ankit Jindal, Dr. Valli Kiran and Dr. Ashwin Naik for their guidance and content on the mental wellness section, Arvind Sivaramakrishnan for his encouragement and insights, and Dr. Anoop Amarnath for helping me understand the confluence of technology and medicine.

To all the contributors and authors at Healthcare India, thank you. A big thank you Ganesh Acharya who has been guiding Healthcare India with media and web related activities.

Dr. Vikram Venkateswaran
Bangalore, 6.12.2020

Foreword

"Own Your Health"- what an apt topic in today's context. I want to keep this text. With the ongoing Covid pandemic raging like wildfire and beating down on the population, bringing the global medical fraternity to its knees, the one thing that everyone is talking about is building immunity. And how does one do it? Is it that I consume few tablets, a couple of injections and lo and behold – I am immune magically? No Immunity is built up over years through systemic care and nurture of the body. The food we take, the physical exercises and the yoga we do, the clean environment that we live in: all have a part to play.

Vikram has beautifully segregated the topics into three parts and each of these parts have a significant role to play in our collective well-being.

As an individual ensure that you consume a healthy, well-balanced diet with lots of vegetables and fruits. Avoid, the use of tobacco, alcohol or drugs, maintain an exercise regimen of at least 45 min a day, avoid mood swings and anger, rest enough, protect yourself against the weather and see your health-care provider if you think something may be wrong: don't self-medicate. My ex-boss would talk about the 8*8*8 principle (drink 8 glasses of water, 8 hours of sleep and 8 kms of walk). He used to practice it religiously and it really kept him in good stead. A routine executive check-up can help identify potential life threatening situations and help with early interventions, thereby resulting in very positive outcomes.

From an industry perspective, digital technologies are turning the industry on its head and redefining the rules of the game. It will help transform unsustainable healthcare systems into sustainable ones, bring in trust and transparency between medical professionals and patients, provide cheaper, faster and more effective solutions for diseases – technologies can help win the battle for us against cancer, AIDS or Ebola – and could simply lead to healthier individuals living in healthier communities. As a medical futurist says, "One has to be a master of his own house, so it is worth starting "the future" with the betterment of our own health through digital technologies, as well as changing our own attitude towards the concept of health, medicine and healthcare." The onus is on us to take advantage of these developments and keep our body and mind fit and healthy.

The Government, too has a significant role to play in the wellbeing of the individual as also the community at large. The areas of public health responsibility include (1) assuring an adequate local public health infrastructure, (2) promoting healthy communities and healthy behaviours, (3) arresting and preventing the spread of communicable disease, (4) protecting against environmental health hazards, (5) shoring up emergency response systems, and (6) assuring health services for all the population.

As Jason Crandall says "The nature of yoga is to shine the light of awareness into the darkest corners of the body." I would end with the following:

सर्वे भवन्तु सुखिनःसर्वे सन्तु निरामयाः।सर्वे भद्राणि पश्यन्तु मा कश्चिद्दुदखभाग्भवेत् ॥

sarve bhavantu sukhinaH, sarve santu nirAmayAH,sarve bhadrANi pashyantu, mA kashchid_duHkha-bhAg-bhavet.

All should/must be happy, be healthy, see good; may no one have a sorrow in heart. Be healthy, stay happy, stay blessed.

Regards
Ravi Ramaswamy
CEO, RV Consultants

Introduction

In late 2017 I was on the tennis courts on a sunny morning in Bangalore where a strange phenomenon occurred. While returning my partner's serve, I felt that the strength in my arms had somehow disappeared. I was trying to hit hard but the ball was hardly crossing the net.

An instructor was noticing this, and he came over and started giving me some instructions on how to return faster and harder. While he was focusing on my hand rotation and getting my centre of gravity below the ball, the returns kept getting weaker and weaker.

In desperation, I finally quit the session, went home and told my wife what had happened. She felt that maybe it was a recurrence of my tennis elbow, which had been plaguing me for some time in the past. I have been playing tennis since 1985 and many times over the years, I have suffered from 'tennis elbow'.

So I went to a sports specialist, an Orthopaedecian who specialized in sports injuries. He took one look at me and asked, when was the last time I got my vitamin D levels tested. I was taken aback because Orthopedicians normally don't ask such a question. But I had been testing my vitamin D levels regularly for the past many years and I shared my results. He then asked, "Have you also tested your vitamin B 12 levels?". As someone who consumes milk products regularly, I was surprised by that question. "I don't think vitamin B 12 is an issue, because I consume milk and paneer regularly and both are important sources of Vitamin B 12", I said. He said I was suffering from a Vitamin B 12 deficiency that was manifesting itself as muscle weakness in my arms, especially around the wrists and forearms - both of which are essential to tennis.

I spent the next three weeks, taking shots for vitamin B 12. What was fascinating is that he did not want me to do a blood test to confirm whether I had vitamin B 12 deficiency. Over the period of three weeks, my arm strength improved significantly and the weakness that I felt in my legs was gone. But it exposed me to the fact that I knew so little about my own body.

Many of us tend to make a lot of assumptions about our health based on our diet, genetics and our medical history, but sometimes forget that simple issues like a vitamin deficiency can cause a major concern. My doctor had not only pointed this out, but had also educated me on the importance of monitoring vital health parameters. Since that day, I have added Vitamin B 12 to the list of parameters that I regularly check for.

How many of us monitor our health regularly? What parameters do we check for? How much do we understand the effect that our actions can have on our bodies?

I am a qualified doctor who practiced for six years before pursuing an MBA to work with healthcare systems globally.

Despite all the information I had and access to experts that I possessed, I still struggled with a lot of my health parameters. I often estimated my health parameters based on my memory, or on my assumptions, rather than monitoring parameters regularly by collecting data and developing a system of accurate and systematic reporting.

My experiences in doing this prompted me to share some best practices with others. This book is my effort to help you to monitor your health and detect issues that can become serious concerns.

The incidents that I describe in the later pages, have affected me, my friends and family. I share some examples of how you can manage these incidents (should you experience them) with a combination of doctors, technology applications on your smart phone and a little help from the internet.

This book is not a substitute for a doctor, not does it undermine the medical community.

The objective, is to avoid unnecessary medication and hospitalization, and to ensure that your physical and mental wellbeing is in your hands, so doctors can heal those who really need their help with serious ailments.

Can I realistically care for my health? The answer is yes, In fact in my experience, you are the only one who can own your health.

No one knows you better than you yourself. No matter how hard somebody else tries, they may never be able to get to the depth of your understanding of your senses, your values, your customs, your personality, what your soul wants, and what your body wants to tell you.

For the same reason, you can't take charge of someone's health.

Of course, should your body encounter something different, you must seek medical help to understand the issue and watch out for symptoms in the future.

I want to thank you for purchasing this book. I know you had a lot of choices, to spend your time and money, which are very valuable. By investing in this book, I hope you are able to appreciate the wonderful system that the human body is and get closer to yours.

Own Your Health.

Dr. Vikram Venkateswaran

To Treat is good, To Prevent is better – Own Your Health

Since my childhood, I remember a board hung in my mother's clinic in the 1980's that said

"I treat, he cures"

As a dentist she spent a lot of time with patients those days - both in her practice and the rural medical centre she used to visit. She often told me that while giving the treatment was in her hands, the patient needed to think positively and own his health to be cured. I grew up with that philosophy.

"Sarvojana Sukhino Bhavantu" - This wisdom from the Vedas means "Let everyone be happy."

Happiness is the goal of all human beings and good health is one of the foundations of happiness.

Our health is in our hands. We have the power to manage it and today we have the tools to help us do that effectively. We have access to the most modern technologies and cloud based platforms to preserve information. Mobile applications can be used to track our workout, including activities like walking and practices like Yoga.

Yet, health tends to be the most neglected part of our lives. Why is this?

Unless one is afflicted with a lifestyle or lifelong ailment since childhood, the chances are he/she has a very reactive approach to healthcare. Most of us pop a pill (generic mostly, which costs next to nothing) when we are diagnosed with fever, aches, and other issues.

Many in rural India will use home grown remedies for treating minor ailments. The notion of systematically preventing disease through lifestyle changes doesn't strike us, until it is too late. This is when we turn to hospitalisation or lifelong treatment.

This attitude is also reflected in the public health spending by various governments in India. An analysis of select 2014 election manifestos indicates that we may be woefully behind on the path to a more comprehensive health plan for citizens. The bulk of healthcare in India - prevention, treatment and care - remains in the hands of medical practitioners.

But being a doctor, I know that most of us in the community would like patients to manage their health beyond a point. Emergencies, rare diseases, infections and palliative care (care for the terminally ill) are all the areas where doctors would like to spend their time and expertise. Also the doctor patient ratio in India is very poor, so the more you can take care of your health the better it is for our healthcare system.

In line with that this book has three sections.

Section 1 – The Individual- How you can own your health

Section 2- The Healthcare Industry- What the industry is doing to help you take charge of your Health? This section covers new procedures, technology and therapies that the industry is working with that can help you.

Section 3- The Government -What is the government doing to help you maintain your health?

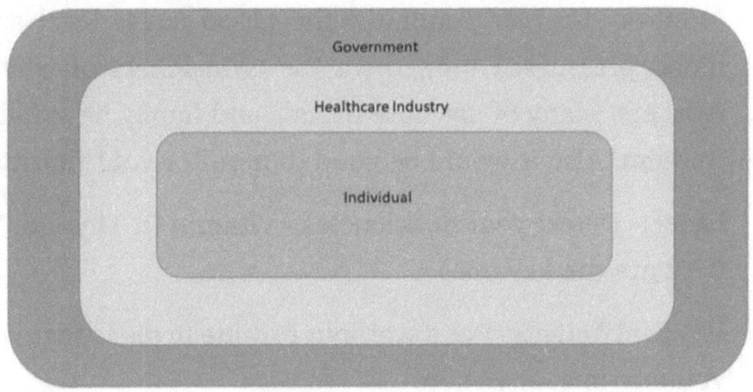

Diagram 1 The Healthcare Ecosystem as it impacts the individual

The structure above gives you a sense of where you stand with regards to the ecosystem. Though your health depends on you, the industry and the government do have a big impact on your health as well.

How can you own your health? The below sample framework can help you get started with your self-care journey. I would recommend that you take out your diary or a note book and draw this framework there. Towards the end of the section we will fill this with my recommendations. You can also modify this based on your personal need.

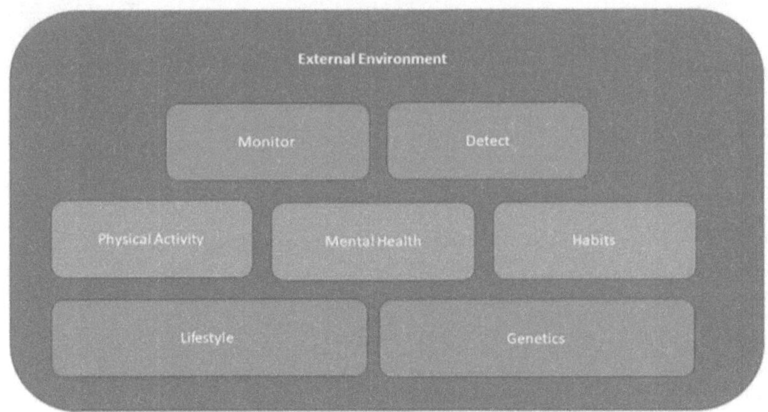

Diagram 2 The Own Your Health Framework

- Monitor- Regularly monitor the blood sugar level and your blood pressure. I term them the twin killers of white-collar workers. Many of my close friends and family have fallen prey to them. Also it would be good to monitor your nutrition

- Detect- Detect your deficiencies - Vitamin D, Thyroid, Vitamin B 12 are the key ones

- Physical Activity- Put a workout routine in place that works for you anytime, anywhere

- Mental Health – Keep a healthy mind, identify red flags for mental issues

- Habits- Watch your alcohol levels and smoking, also watch the usual suspects like salt and sugar consumption.

- Lifestyle – Introduce practices like Yoga and Ayurveda

- Genetics- Know more about your genes and what ailments you can be pre-disposed to.

For most of these areas, one can use a smartphone to monitor progress. The cases discussed in the coming pages will tell you how.

SECTION 1
Your Health

The twin killers of white-collar workers – Part 1 – Diabetes

In January of 2018, I lost my mother. Of all the things that have happened to me that were painful or sad, this was probably the worst. It left a hole in my life that no one or nothing can ever fill. My mother was a strong lady and a pillar of strength for me. But the last five years were not kind to her. She had suffered two fractures, one bypass and kidney issues. All this was courtesy of a foundational lifestyle condition that weakened her daily.

That condition was Diabetes.

Diabetes is a condition, not a disease, and stems from the inability of the body to regulate the sugar in the blood. As diabetes is a multi-factor condition, it is difficult to pin it to one reason or factor. But one of the causative factors is genetics. My mother had diabetes and so did my grandmother. Interestingly my great grandfather had diabetes too. So in a way I am genetically predisposed to it. However, there are a few things that might still work in my favour namely

- The genes I inherited from my fathers' side

- Diet and nutrition,

- Fitness and Mental Health

India has been called the "Diabetes Capital of the World" in recent times and over 50-60 million people suffer from Type-2 diabetes.

Obesity, aging population, leading a sedentary life and unhealthy diet enhance the chances for this type of diabetes to develop.

Keep your eyes open for these major symptoms of diabetes

High blood glucose level is the major symptom of diabetes. This, in turn, happens because of less or no production of insulin. The body's inability to accept insulin can also be the case that gives rise to diabetes. You must visit the doctor immediately if you come across any of these symptoms mentioned below.

- More urges to use the bathroom

- Greater fatigue and hunger tendencies

- Dry mouth

- Unusual thirst

- Blurred vision

- Itchy skin

- Slow wound healing

- Leg numbness and infection

- Infection of the skin

Is it possible to prevent diabetes?

Unfortunately, gestational diabetes (during pregnancy) and Type 1 diabetes (in children) cannot be prevented. But the risks associated with it can be controlled and managed with a healthy lifestyle, the right medication, and an effective dietary plan.

But it is possible to prevent type 2 diabetes

According to the various clinical trials all across the globe, a structured healthy diet and an active lifestyle can overcome genetic factors and prevent the onset of Type 2 diabetes.

Can diabetes be cured?

No! Diabetes cannot be completely cured. But it can be controlled and managed to a great extent.

In order to control diabetes, you need a comprehensive diabetes treatment plan by an expert doctor. It requires a balance of a planned diet, exercise and medication. It should incorporate constant blood glucose level monitoring followed by routine check-ups by nutritionist, orthopaedecian, gynaecologist, ophthalmologist as well as an endocrinologist.

Measures to control diabetes

Controlling your diabetes requires a lot of patience, meticulous observation, and unfailing dedication to keep the blood sugar level as close to the normal level as possible. Some suggestions are mentioned below.

- **Regulate your carbohydrate intake** –Carbohydrates affect your blood glucose level and that is why you should keep track of the amount that you ingest. Per meal, women require 35-45 grams while men require 45-60 grams of carbohydrates.

- **Take exercise as your medicine** – This should be followed religiously if you have diabetes. You should dedicate a minimum of 150 minutes to working out every week. This can be divided into smaller chunks like 30 minutes each day for five days every week. Just walking, running or cycling can be sufficient. Ask your health coach or a gym instructor for an exercise plan or you can do some research and build a plan for yourself. It is best to keep changing the exercise plan as the mind has a habit of getting used to the exercise and may not respond over time. We will discuss physical activity in detail in the subsequent pages. We will also discuss how there are fitness apps that are available to help you take care of your workout regimen.

- **Never miss your routine check-ups with your team of doctors** – Diabetes is an ailment that involves your complete body. That is why, you should build a dream team of physicians that include your doctor, nurse, dentist, nutritionist, orthopaedecian and many others and go for regular check-ups.

- **Spot check your sugar level** – It is true that you and your doctor will check your sugar level on a regular basis but you should always check on top of that. Spot checking your blood glucose level is of utmost significance for any diabetic so that apt measures can be taken on time before it is too late. For that, you must always carry a quality glucometer from a reputed brand so that you can regularly check your level of blood glucose and gain better control of your condition. I use a glucometer from Dr. Morepen Labs, that comes with the Diabetes pen and the strips.

- **Keep a Track of Your Numbers** – Just checking the blood sugar levels is not enough when you suffer from diabetes as this disease affects your entire body. You need to keep a track of your blood pressure, weight as well as your cholesterol level. Only then you can live a risk-free life.

Monitoring your sugar levels – HbA1c

Now this section might seem slightly technical but it is a very critical part of your defence against diabetes. Anyone who has taken science till 9th standard should be familiar with this concept. The average life of the Red Blood Cell (RBC), is around 120 days. With an estimated half-life of 2-3 months, it is a good indication of the overall health of the individual. Glucose molecules in the blood combine with haemoglobin, and through this glycation form a Ketoamine that is stable and can be used as a measure of the glucose in the blood. Since 1970's HbA1c measures have been recommended as a standard of care for diabetes management.

Why is this a better measure than the traditional fasting and Post-Prandial measures (PP)?

1.   Firstly, measuring HbA1c gives us the story of the blood sugar levels for 90 days. So it not a point in time investigation rather it's a holistic view of the system.

2.   It is human tendency to cheat if we know that a blood sugar test is looming. I have seen my mother do that many times and there are dietary adjustments made just before the test that can give us a false negative.

3.   Thirdly the test does not require any fasting or dietary restrictions, hence the compliance is better.

All this is documented in research published by Sherwani Et All in the US Library of Public Medicine.

The HbA1c cannot be tested through a home glucometer, that means you have to get it tested in a lab. While these are great reasons to conduct the test, the key to the test is to go to an accredited lab. Always insist on choosing a NABL (National Accreditation Board for Testing and Calibration Laboratories) accredited lab.

Finally, talk to your doctor on why you should consider mapping this level. I have been doing my tests over a period of time and last few months' results are shown below. These tests have given my physician a good indication as to why I need more aggressive intervention.

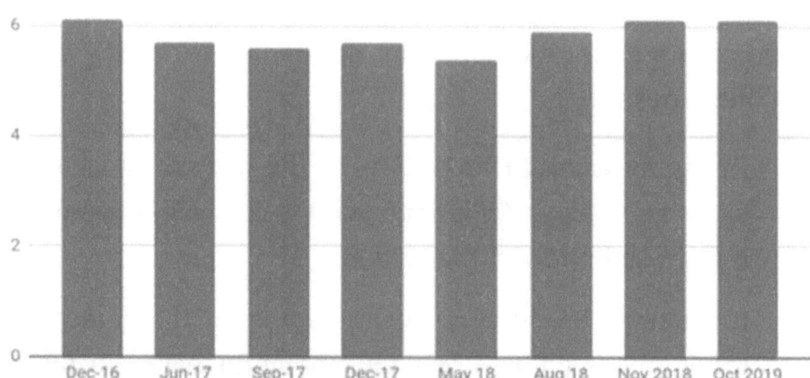

Diagram 3 My HbA1c levels from 2016 to 2019, as you can see I have tried to keep it in the range of 6 and below

Below is the table to keep track of your hbA1c Levels

HbA1c	mmol/mol	%
Normal	Below 42 mmol/mol	Below 6.0%
Prediabetes	42 to 47 mmol/mol	6.0% to 6.4%
Diabetes	48 mmol/mol or over	6.5% or over

Diagram 4 The levels of HbA1c for Normal, Prediabetes and Diabetes

Having mostly kept it below 6% I have maintained my sugar levels in the no Diabetes range. But of course that can change hence the need to keep track of these levels regularly. Now let's look at another friend that combines well with Diabetes to create a foundation for more diseases-hypertension.

The twin killers of white-collar workers – Part 2 – Hypertension

I used to work with an advertising executive, let us call him Prakash. An MBA from a premier institute, he fit the stereotype of a successful corporate executive. One Wednesday morning he was driving to work. He was stuck in a traffic jam in the peak hour but his mind was somewhere else. The week had been a rough one with three client deliverables due, and his team was struggling to meet them. As he was sitting in the car and planning his day, he felt his head spin and he could not see very clearly. He blinked his eyes and rubbed his eye lids, hoping it was just dryness in his contact lenses aggravated by the car's air conditioning.

Soon he was experiencing difficulty in breathing. Felling nauseous, he rolled down his windows and tried to loosen his shirt. He started sweating profusely and there was a shooting pain through his temples. Prakash knew he was in trouble and had the common sense to call out to the car next to him for help. A passer-by notified the traffic police and a good samaritan rung up the ambulance service. Prakash had little recollection of what happened next, but he was saved in time by the emergency services who rushed him to the nearest hospital.

What Prakash experienced was a spike in his blood pressure that can be fatal. If not controlled, it can lead to heart failure and ischaemic heart disease, stroke, and renal failure. Luckily for him it was managed properly and he was restored to normal life and has since then managed his blood pressure well. A few months later, Prakash took a break from work and opted for a less demanding role. While I was happy to see

Prakash moving on with his life, I knew many more who were not so lucky.

According to statistics almost one in three people in urban India are hypertensive. The most dangerous part of this condition is that it is non-symptomatic. So there is no warning before a spike in blood pressure levels. This means one needs to monitor and manage their blood pressure. Normal blood pressure is 120-130/80 mm Hg. Any reading above 140/80 mm Hg can be considered hypertensive, particularly a rise in the lower levels can be more dangerous and a reading above 85 should be taken seriously.

Hypertension can also increase the risk of development of Cardio Vascular Disease.

Management of Hypertension

The philosophy of this book is "Prevention is better than Cure". In case of Hypertension it is the only way to handle the condition. In Prakash's case his family doctor advised him to do the following

1. Lifestyle changes – Making healthy lifestyle changes can help improve as well as reverse the condition. These include eating fresh food, avoiding junk food, sleeping and waking up on time.

2. Reduce Weight -Achieving one's ideal weight is the best treatment for high blood pressure. Blood pressure tends to rise as body weight increases. To lose weight, it is best to work eat healthy, maintain portion control and be physically active. Keeping a watch on your BMI (Body mass index) and WC(Waist circumference) is important. (A waist measurement of 90 cms or above for (Asian) men and 80 cm or above for Asian (Women) poses a significant health risk).

3. To Quit or reduce smoking- Smoking causes a constriction of the blood vessels leading to a temporary increase in the blood pressure, over a period of time this can prove fatal. We shall discuss this in the coming pages in more detail.

4. Reduce dietary salt intake - Salt can be a very dangerous ingredient for those with high blood pressure. Again salt increases the osmotic pressure in the blood leading to increased pressure. Again we shall discuss salt in more details in subsequent pages.

5. Reduce alcohol consumption- Again another habit we need to monitor. We will discuss more about that later

6. Follow de-stressing techniques such as meditation, yoga and breathing exercises. Regularly spend time amidst nature and near plants.

Should all these changes still leave you at the risk of hypertension, the doctors would likely recommend Anti-Hypertensive drugs to control the condition. It is very important that one does not self-medicate but seek and follow the advice of the physician.

Typically, a doctor would check for the following parameters prior to prescribing medication.

Key Investigations	Normal Range
Blood Pressure	Systolic/Diastolic range of 120-130/80 mm Hg (The Diastolic number is more critical)
Blood Sugar	100 or less than 100 mg/dl (Fasting)
HbA1c	5.6-6 % (Average of 120 days or life of RBC)

Diagram 5 Key parameters that you need to monitor, the blood sugar we have discussed earlier, blood pressure check is important, HbA1c is important as well

Other checks that may be prescribed include

Lipid Profile	Range
Total Cholesterol	< 200 mg/dL
Triglycerides	<150 mg/dL
HDL Cholesterol	Male: <40 mg/dL, Female: <50 mg/dL
LDL Cholesterol	< 100 mg/dL
VLDL Cholesterol	< 30 mg/dL

Diagram 6 Lipid and Cholesterol have a huge impact on the blood pressure, important to keep these parameters in check

All checks should be conducted following a doctor's prescription and from authorized laboratories only. For general blood pressure monitoring I have an Omron Blood Pressure monitor at home. I use it regularly and over a period of time, I have been able to see a link between headaches or stress and high blood pressure.

To ascertain your pre-disposition to hypertension, you may look for the following signs

- Family history of Hypertension - Most important factor, in my case I have a history of hypertension from my father's side, incidentally my paternal grandmother lost her life to hypertension.

- High BMI and accumulation of fat in the abdomen area

- Habits like Smoking and Alcohol

Now let's look at some key factors that you need to monitor on a regular basis, let's start with what you eat.

Tracking your nutrition

How often do you check packaging of processed food items (like jams, chips, ready to cook or eat meals) for their nutritional value? Most people usually toss these items in the shopping cart without thinking twice about what they are about to consume.

Given that Indian food is generally high on carbohydrates and there is a preference for junk foods, the nutritional value of a meal tends to be diluted. Further, the required daily nutrient intake too can suffer leading to various lifestyle disorders such as diabetes and hypertension.

You are what you eat is a common adage.

The rule of thumb that I follow is - eat what my forefathers have eaten. As a rule, I stay away from fancy diets, like Mediterranean food or Keto Diet etc. My diet is strictly vegetarian and mostly South Indian.

I also avoid packaged food for its high salt and sugar content. Salt and sugar are good preservatives but can wreak havoc with calories as well as increase water retention, if consumed in large quantities. (Our ancestors used limited helpings/ servings of preserved foods like pickles, sweets, chutneys, papads and jams in their meal, preferring to use them as accompaniments and not the main course.)

The awareness of nutrient intake and calorie count is relatively low in India because traditional meals were designed to enable us to undertake traditional labour - manual work that did not allow for long periods of sedentary work. Further, food was seasonal and cooked in a manner to preserve nutrients and give us the strength to carry out our daily chores. Sweets were an indulgence and restricted to festivals and important days.

Today in urban India, our lifestyles are very different and our food habits have changed, without understanding how this can impact our health, particularly the calories we consume and the nutrition we gain.

Here is where technology can come to the rescue. Thanks to our smart phones now, we have access to many mobile applications that can track our nutrition.

I personally use HealthifyMe, a mobile app that has a good database of Indian regional foods and can quantify calories in them.

Of the many features in this app, the one that I use is having the calories instantly counted based on a picture of the food item. Thanks to an in-house nutritionist, the meal is analysed, and feedback is provided on the estimated calories and the macro-nutrient values. The company also has an in-house tool, built from the National Institute of Nutrition's database, to calculate the nutrition value of any food based solely on its ingredients and the cooking procedure. The nutritionists hired by the company are associated with medical establishments such as Medanta, Apollo and Manipal hospitals. They can provide consultations to patients from cardiology, endocrinology and preventive health centers, and are selected on the basis of their clinical experience and elaborate case studies of patients.

If you are looking for weight loss assistance, the app can also build a program designed to suit your physical, medical and motivational levels. All the fitness experts on the App are ACE certified and work full-time with the company. The app also has psychologists to help customers stay motivated during their journey.

I have been using this application for the last many months. The calorie counts of some of the food that I thought was 'healthy' was surprisingly high. As a doctor, if I was unaware, then you can imagine what the common Indian goes through daily, by unknowingly consuming food that might affect his health in the future.

While I have used HealthifyMe, there are other trackers that I have used in the past that can also be effective.

1.	My fitness plan Calorie Counter- From Under Armour

2.	Calorie Counter

3.	Nutrition Data Indian Food

Why use an app?

Well it is important to keep a record of what you have consumed otherwise you tend to go with memory and the mind always plays a trick on you. Not keeping records is what causes many fitness programs to fail and diet is an important part of the regimen.

My suggestion is to download the apps, don't cheat and see which one works for you. But while we monitor so many parameters how do you detect a deficiency? The next chapter outlines some parameters to consider. Let's look at the first one Vitamin D.

There is no sunshine when Vitamin D is gone

Some time ago my wife had hired a trainer to help her with her fitness. I was curious how this would work and hence I also decided to work with the same trainer for my fitness journey.

I am no stranger to workouts, and I had been leveraging trainers before in the various gyms that I had been a member with. But this was different. As my training started the first thing I remember was that there was intense pain in my muscles and joints. Despite painkillers, the pain would not go away. The trainer kept telling me that it was a matter of time and things would improve. She even brought in another trainer, who helped me with some stretching exercises. But when things got worse, I had to consult my family physician. One look at me, he asked, "When was the last time you checked your Vitamin D levels?". That started a quest for monitoring my Vitamin D levels, which continues till this day.

Vitamin D deficiency symptoms

Vitamin D is produced by the body due to exposure to sunlight light. It is an important element that a human body requires. In 2010, the Institute of Medicine (IOM) issued a report based on a lengthy examination of data on Vitamin D levels by a group of experts. To sum up, they estimated that a vitamin D level of 20 mg/mL or higher was adequate for good bone health, and subsequently, a level below that was considered a vitamin D deficiency.

Below are the charts I have kept for my Vitamin D Levels. As you can see I started with a deficiency around 11 and now have managed to keep myself above the 20 mark for the last 5 years.

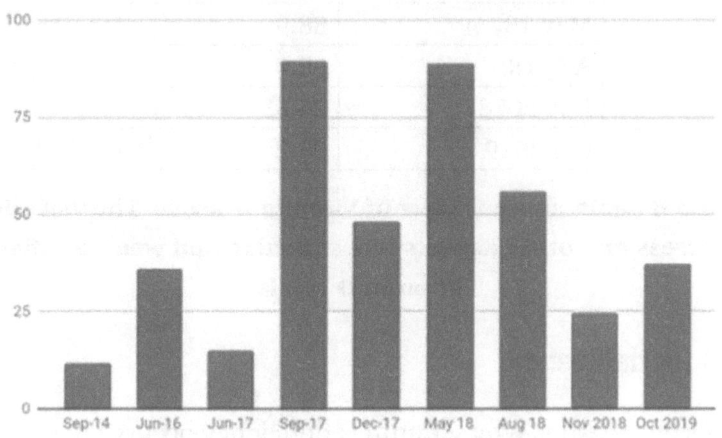

Diagram 7 Since 2014 I have tracked my Vitamin D levels, as you can make out this is a recurring battle where the levels have dropped to dangerous levels like in 2017 June

As you can see, from my experience with the trainer in September 2014 where my levels were at 11.8, I have tried to maintain a higher level. But in June 2017 again my levels fell to 15. Why this happened is difficult to say as I was standing in the sun regularly. But then, a city like Bangalore tends to not have as much sun as a city like say Chennai. Also, one's capacity to absorb sunlight is also an important factor in Vitamin D levels. So unless one constantly monitors Vitamin D levels, it is not possible to maintain the requisite levels of over 20 mg/mL.

Date	Levels(ng/dl)
Sep-14	11.8
Jun-16	36.1
Jun-17	15.07
Sep-17	89.5
Dec-17	48.15
May 18	88.9
Aug 18	55.9
Nov 2018	24.58
Oct 2019	37.2

Diagram 8 Again another view of Vitamin D levels. The variation in levels, stress and other aspects like sunshine and weather affects the Vitamin D levels

Reasons for deficiency

The numerous reasons why vitamin D deficiency occurs are given below.

1. Sedentary lifestyle, mostly spent indoors

2. Less exposure to direct sunlight

3. Extensive use of sunblock and sunscreen

4. Limited absorption of vitamin D.

5. Hereditary factors

Key symptoms of Vitamin D deficiency

Weakness and pain: The weakness of bones and muscles is the first sign that there might be a problem. Weak bones are feature of vitamin D deficiency; however, they can also generally occur at an early age or older age. Other symptoms include muscle cramps, weakness and nagging pain after exercise or a walk.

Obesity: Individuals who are obese tend to show signs of lower vitamin D levels.

Feeling Low: It is difficult to explain, but lack of Vitamin D has been linked to subclinical depression. This often leads to mood swings and lethargy.

Other symptoms: Some other signs are a knock-kneed appearance, low blood calcium levels, high blood pressure levels

So what do you do if you experience any of these symptoms? In my opinion you could follow the below steps.

1. Visit a doctor- Please visit a doctor or set up a telemedicine consultation. This is just to ensure that the symptoms you have are in line with Vitamin D deficiency. Please do not self-medicate.

2. Check your Vitamin D Levels regularly from a NABL certified Lab.

3. Plan for at least 30 minutes of outdoor activity daily especially in the morning- Walking, Jogging or just stretching in the park can be helpful. Avoid standing in the hot sun between 9:00 am and 5:00 pm, as intense rays of sun may do more damage than enhancing Vitamin D production.

4. Keep a record of your Vitamin D levels

5. Eat foods rich in Vitamin D- Almonds, Spinach, Milk are some of the common foods that we find in India that can help increase Vitamin D levels.

Now let me introduce you to another parameter that you may want to keep in mind as you go along with journey.

Into the danger zone with thyroid

During Medical College, when I first saw the outline of the thyroid gland, I was pretty surprised by its size and its position. It is a very small butterfly shaped gland that works very closely with the pituitary gland. Together they control almost every hormone that is secreted in the human body. Hyperthyroidism is a result of over activity of the gland, whereas hypothyroidism is the reverse condition.

In India, among the white collar workforce, one will likely find many cases of hypothyroidism or an underactive thyroid.

The first thing you will notice about hypothyroidism is fatigue. You will feel very tired, without having exercised or done anything physically exerting and may experience pain, stiffness or swelling in your joints. The daily office routine of just staring at a desk and a computer can be enough to tire you out. The second symptom is sensitivity to cold. You will feel colder than usual and even a 20 degree' centigrade weather would see you put on your jacket. Hypothyroidism also leads to constipation and dry skin. Lastly, unexplained weight gain, even if you are controlling your diet and eating healthy.

In some cases, thinning of hair or unusual hair loss is also attributed to hypothyroidism.

So, what causes all these issues?

The most common cause is stress and a sedentary lifestyle. The thyroid gland produces two main hormones. One is tri iodothyronine, or T3, and the other is called thyroxin or T4.

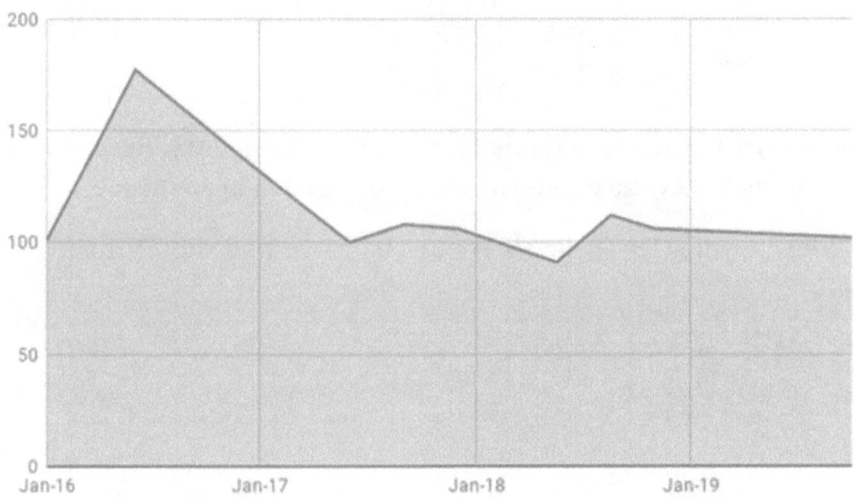

Diagram 9 T3 levels that I have been monitoring after the brief spike in 2016, mostly I have kept it at about 100 levels

These two hormones in combination with the thyroid stimulating hormone (TSH) has an enormous impact on your metabolic rate. They also control a lot of vital body functions like your temperature, heart rate. When these hormones are not produced in adequate numbers (due to stress or limited physical activity), we experience hypo or hyperthyroidism. Below is a chart showing how my thyroid levels have fluctuated over the years.

My T3 Triiodothyronine levels from January 2016- October 2019

T3		
	Jan-16	101
	Jun-16	177
	Jun-17	100
	Sep-17	108

(Contd.)

T3		
	Dec-17	106
	May 18	91
	Aug 18	112
	Nov 2018	106
	Oct 2019	102

Diagram 10 The T3 Levels from my tests from 2016-2019, despite a brief dip in May 2018, mostly have managed to keep them up

Ideally, your T3 T4 levels should be high, and the TSH should be low.

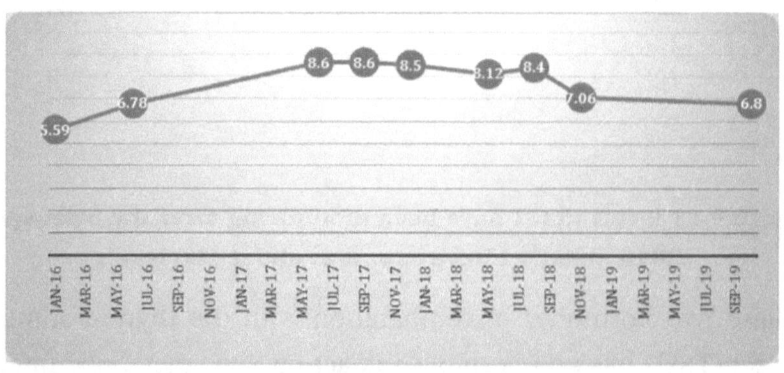

Diagram 11 My T4 levels from 2016-2019 again I have managed to keep them above 6

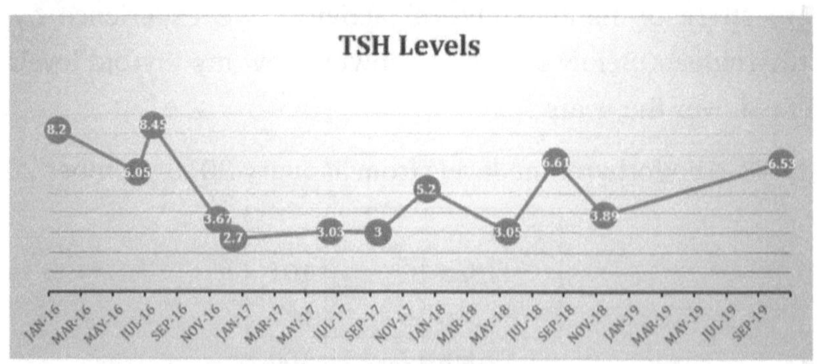

Diagram 12 TSH Levels again lower levels are better, as you can see towards the 2019 again TSH Levels have spiked

So it is important to track them and again you would need to get these levels tested regularly in a NABL accredited Lab.

While Vitamin D and Thyroid formed the bedrock of the detect strategy, the incident at the tennis court that I mentioned in the beginning of the book, led me to add one more element to my testing regimen. That element is Vitamin B 12

The strange case of Vitamin B12

Vitamin B 12 is used in the production of red blood cells that carry oxygen to the different parts of the body. The lack of vitamin B12 causes a deficiency of oxygen, resulting in lack of strength - both to the muscles to and to the mind. It often affects vegetarians, vegans and those who have undergone a weight reduction surgery. In extreme cases it leads to paranoia and depression. The deficiency takes time to build but does impact abruptly and in my case leads to some painful consequences.

Interestingly, Vitamin B 12 is one of the few vitamins that is not made by plants and having a vegetarian diet, or if you're strictly vegan means you could be susceptible to vitamin B12 deficiency. The richest sources of vitamin B 12 include eggs, poultry, and milk. So if you decide to opt for black coffee and do not make up for the milk lost in your diet (like I had done for some time prior to experiencing challenges during a game of tennis), you may end up with a Vitamin B12 deficiency. Some of the symptoms for vitamin b12 deficiency include the following:

- Tingling sensation in your hands or feet.

- Challenges in your gait or balancing yourself on your feet.

- Swollen or inflamed tongue

- Difficulty in remembering things, thinking and reasoning

Interestingly the more we go digital, the more trouble we have with thinking and reasoning due to fatigue. Below is a chart that shows the Vitamin B12 Levels. Should you experience any of the symptoms listed above, and should your doctor prescribe a test, these levels can be useful indicators.

Level	Stage
300-950 Picograms / Millilitre	Normal
300-200 Picograms / Millilitre	Borderline
Below 200 Picograms / Millilitre	Deficiency

Diagram 13 Levels of Vitamin B 12

While a doctor can prescribe a Vitamin B 12 supplement, you may also add milk and milk products to your diet.

You may also take cereals, or bread that come fortified with B12 multivitamin.

As with monitoring other hormone levels, Vitamin B12 should also be monitored at least once in six months.

While most of these parameters are sneaky and hard to detect, there are some obvious areas that we choose to ignore. Speaking of ignoring, one area that we cannot choose to ignore is dental hygiene. It's important to track and to ensure that it is within the range.

Dental hygiene – smile it increases your health value

I have spent almost all my life in close proximity of dentistry. My mother was a practising dentist and so was I. I have learnt as a child and later professionally, the importance of dental care in our overall health.

Digestion begins from the mouth. What you put in your mouth and how it gets digested determines your overall health.

If you don't have proper dental hygiene, and you're not careful about maintaining your teeth, then your overall health can suffer. Specifically, poor dental hygiene by itself can result in a host of issues that can interfere with your health.

Many times systemic issues like hypertension and diabetes, and even cardiovascular diseases manifest themselves in the mouth. The swelling of gums could be as a sign of hypertension. Sometimes the unnecessary bleeding from the gums and its inability to stop soon, could be due to diabetic conditions or high sugar levels.

Stress and psychological changes are also manifested in the mouth, whether it is the erosion of teeth due to acidity or clenching or grinding of teeth in tense moments. There is a condition called bruxism where the individual involuntarily clenches his teeth leading to pain in the jaws and wearing down of the teeth.

How can you maintain dental hygiene?

It is a good practice to gently brush your teeth twice a day using a toothbrush and toothpaste. There are a couple of techniques for brushing but a safe option is the circular technique (or the modified bass technique) in which you brush your teeth up and down in a circle (as opposed to side to side).

A couple of other remedies to try at least once a week is to gargle. Salt is a great disinfectant and gargling your teeth using a little salt and warm water once a week can keep your mouth healthy. One of the precautions to COVID-19 has also been gargling daily, because any virus entering your throat can be neutralised with saltwater gargles.

In case of any pain or discomfort in your teeth, do not put it off. Immediately seek a dentist's help. A common issue among some patients is impaction – or where the molar teeth are not straight due to the lack of space in the jaw. They slant to one side leading to gum infections and caries. Best to have them checked regularly and to take action to prevent any serious issues at a later stage.

Avoid using toothpicks and sharp objects to dislodge food stuck to the teeth or address irritation in gums. If your food is getting stuck in your teeth, it is most likely because of some infection or inflammation in your gums.

The other interesting observation I have is the decision that many people make to extract a tooth if there is a cavity on them. The teeth are very important for your digestion and losing a tooth early is not a good idea. Try seeing if a root canal or a restorative surgery is possible on the tooth. Teeth are also important for our speech and holding the shape of the face.

I receive a lot of questions on teeth whitening. Whitening comes with its own set of challenges. It is important to understand why you would want to use whitening techniques before getting started.

Visit your dentist once in six months for an examination of the mouth and a regular cleaning.

Don't take any dental ailment lightly. If you have a pain in your teeth or swelling in your gums, don't try home remedies but reach out to a dentist. If your teeth are key to digestion, then your eyes are your windows to the world.

Eyes – now I see you

One of the biggest casualties of the modern digitized living are our eyes. With greater screen time and compelling content, we often end up blinking less, increasing the dryness in our eyes. On a regular basis one should ideally blink 10-12 times a minute, but now that has reduced by half. As a result, our eyes feel the strain demonstrated by itchiness and heaviness.

Prolonged screen time can result in soreness of the eyes. So what can you do?

Safeguarding your eyes

Consciously blink more to enable natural secretion of tears.

While working on a laptop or watching TV, ensure that the screen brightness levels are adjusted to suit your eyes. Very bright screens tend to strain the eyes faster, whereas very low lit screens also put strain on the eyes.

- Opt for zero power anti-glare glasses which reduces strain and can help prolong working hours.

- Ensure you are sitting in a well-lit spot while working. If the ambient lighting the room is good, the eyes adjust faster to the brightness with less strain.

- If there is dryness, itchiness and watering of the eyes, please consult an ophthalmologist. If you are seeing the doctor for the first time, physical consultation may be better but telemedicine can be used for subsequent meetings.

To prevent dryness in the eyes, there are two specific things that you can do.

The first is the 20-20-20 formula. This is pretty common sense but was introduced to me by my good friend and ophthalmologist Dr. Abhiyan Kumar. This involves looking at an object that is 20 feet away for 20 seconds, every 20 minutes that you look at a screen. This can relax the eye muscles and help them focus better.

20 Seconds – Duration	Look away
20 Feet – Distance	Distance from you
20 Minutes – Screen time	Of Screen Time

Diagram 14 The 20-20-20 formula is a good hack to reduce the strain on the eyes

On similar lines, eye exercises prescribed in Yoga can also be helpful.

The second approach to improve the lubrication of the eye is by consuming Omega 3 capsules that are available as supplements. While these can be bought over the counter at a pharmacy, it is advisable to seek a prescription from the doctor.

In adverse cases, you can try lubricating eye drops, upon your doctor's advice. Please note that these drops have to be used within a month once opened and should not be shared - even among family members.

Despite these measures should the itching persist, please consult a doctor.

Talking of eye soreness reminds me of an incident in 2017.

I had developed an allergy in my eyes, which made me extremely sensitive to bright light. This made it difficult for me to work on the computers as the glare of the display caused tremendous discomfort. I reached out to many friends, colleagues and even so called "IT experts" for a solution, but to my dismay I did not find any. Eventually,

I succumbed to the situation and decided to wear shades to protect my eyes from the glare. However, the solution to my work problem emerged from my colleague Ankit Jindal, who has vision disability.

He guided me to the considerably basic but an extremely useful feature that he has been using for over a decade and is a part of all computers shipped with Windows operating system. I reluctantly tried the "high contrast" option on my computer on his request and I was pleasantly surprised. The feature helped to substantially reduce the glare on the computer screen and provided me the much-needed relief.

This episode led to an interesting dialogue between us where we discussed a range of such technologies that assist people with and without disabilities.

So when I asked Ankit, "what's that one thing that impacted his life the most?"

He exclaims its technology. Ankit says that when he looks back, he can divide his life into two phases, that is life before and after technology.

Ankit grew up in the metropolitan city of Mumbai. He had a very normal, low-key upbringing. He went to school, fought with his younger brother, and had very protective family. It was all very normal, until he was 13, when Ankit was diagnosed with a condition called Retinitis Pigmentosa, also known as RP. He was informed that over a period, he will lose his ability to see, eventually making him blind. Ankit explained that in the next few years, it was not just his vision that went down, but also his aspirations, confidence, and his self-worth. He used to wonder how he would complete his education, especially when it became nearly impossible for him to read books? Will his dream of doing MBA from a premier institute remain just a dream?

Ankit recalled, he would be so envious of his friends and frustrated as they got their fancy laptop and new mobile phones, and were able to do all the wonderful things like chatting, browse the internet, work on assignments and much more. He often wondered, any decent job in the future will require him to use the computers, but he could not operate it. How will he work and earn his livelihood? Would he always have to depend on others for every small and big thing, like managing his currency, travel, watch movies so on and so forth?

The answer to many of these existential questions emerged after being introduced to – technology. And it is just not IT or digital technologies, he was specifically eluding to all products, software, tools, and machines that assist people with disabilities, often referred as assistive technologies or assistive products. People with different disabilities use these technologies to live with independence. Take for instance, hearing aids, wheelchairs, pill organizers, memory aids, etc. have enabled a life of independence, confidence, and dignity. It opened several opportunities to do things which once could have been considered as impossible.

In Ankit's case it was screen-readers. It is a type of assistive technology that enabled him to access first his computer and then his mobile phones. Screen readers are a sophisticated program that converted content on the computer screen including text, file explorer, navigate the menus and much more, into speech output. Among several things, it allowed him to read and learn from content. Throughout his teens, Ankit wanted to read books. And, thanks to the screen-reader, he was finally able to indulge himself. This played a crucial role in doing his MBA from a tier 1 B-school and played foundational for the professional role.

It helped him operate popular office applications that allowed him to create documents, analyse data and make presentations. This increased his employability. With maps on his phone, Ankit was empowered to travel with confidence.

Among other things, he says that he was able to operate his own bank account. He no more had to worry about the signature mismatch and end up in jail for bounced cheques.

This is just one such case-study. A google search can uncover several stories of how assistive technology enables people with disabilities to participate more fully in all aspects of life (home, school, and community) and increases their opportunities for education, social interactions, and potential for meaningful employment. It creates greater independence and control for disabled individuals. All types of people with disabilities whether those having difficulty in hearing, using their limbs, learning and others are benefiting from technology. What is fascinating is that it is just not the erstwhile specialized tools such as wheel-chairs, hearing aids, etc., but also apps / software in our day to day technology like smartphones, smart devices and others that are enabling them to live fulfilling lives.

Unfortunately, not all persons with disabilities have access to assistive technologies. According to WHO less than 10% who need assistive products have access to it. This number could be as low as 5% in emerging countries like India. There is a big gap that needs to be filled to let many populations lead a fulfilling life. There is a need of individuals to be more aware and adopt these solutions.

So while we have come a long way, we do realise that a lot more needs to be done. But take care of your eyes they are your windows to the world. But while monitoring and detecting is good, physical exercise is the best medicine one can get.

Physical activity-fitness: get in the ring

Fitness and I were great friends.

I have been very active in sports all my life. I played tennis ever since I saw Boris Becker beat Kevin Curren in the 1985 Wimbledon finals. I have also played football. Recently I also picked up golf.

But then I lost interest in sports and used to go to the gym regularly. But that also stopped. I was working 12 hours a day and felt it left me with no energy to pursue anything. I just had no drive to go to the sports field or the gym to keep myself fit. At that stage my doctor asked me to pick up an activity of my choice and persist with it.

I tried yoga. I tried hiring a fitness instructor (like I mentioned earlier). I also tried Zumba but nothing worked. I was able to persist with only one physical activity - walking. Covid-19 put an end to that. Just before the lockdown, I had a Cult Fitness membership and was focusing mostly on boxing and football in the sessions.

I ended up sharing the household chores with my wife, and that resulted in my inability to exercise the way I wanted to. I came across a few apps on the phone that were really helpful in maintaining fitness. The best part of using fitness apps is that you need very little space. You can do it in a six by four feet space in your house with just a mat.

Most exercises are freehand and freestyle, which uses your own body weight against you. There are two apps in particular that I want to talk about. The first app is called Seven which has a series of exercises, which you can choose, depending on your body type, your strength level (beginner, intermediate or expert) or exercise type. These exercises are largely based on the high intensity interval training format and can be completed within seven to 10 minutes. If that is not enough for you, you could combine a series of these exercises to stretch your workout to 45 minutes or an hour.

The other app I have used is called Lose Weight. This is also divided into three levels, beginner, intermediate and expert. It provides exercise routines based on circuit/ interval training and involves repetitions that last between seven to 15 minutes. These exercises are intended to induce sweating.

To me, the biggest advantage of using fitness apps like these two has been the ability to track my activity and sync it with other devices/ apps you may be using. Over time, a pattern of how many calories you have burnt and what exercises you have undertaken, can give a sense of what is working for your body and what isn't. For instance, if you are trying to lose weight, then an App can point out previously done exercises so that you may not repeat them. Fitness Apps can also be integrated with your nutrition and diet based apps to get a holistic view of your health.

Fitness Apps may also be paired with wearable devices.

I have used some of them in the past including the Jawbone Up 24 and the Get Active Slim. Both lasted a year and a half before the devices had issues and I had to stop using them. Now I use the Google Fit app on Android and it helps me to keep track of my steps and helps me with fitness goals.

India is the third largest wearables market in the world after the US and China. In 2019 India's wearable market grew by 30%. Interestingly, this market is dominated by ear wear (Blue Tooth Ear Pods) comprising almost 60% of the market. The wrist bands come next and watches make up the last segment.

Finding motivation, time and energy is hard, but it is a lot easier with a fitness tracker. Fitness trackers support fitness and weight reduction by assisting you to attain small victories. They translate all activity into measurable insights and produce analytics that helps you keep track of fitness goals.

Some of the common types of fitness trackers available in the market today include.

1.   Ear Wear- Mostly smart ear phones enabled by Blue Tooth. They play dual functions as ear phones as well as fitness trackers.

2.   Fitness Bands- There are many types of fitness trackers but the most visible ones are wrist devices or fitness bands devoted to total fitness monitoring. Other wearable apparatus can track your health and life, while sleep trackers and physical fitness can help in monitoring your level of fitness. A few wearables also measure your heart beat and monitor cardiac health. But their accuracy can vary.

3.   Pedometers- Basic Pedometers are another resource for monitoring fitness. They are affordable and good for tracking basic exercises like walking.

Below are some interesting characteristics of this market in India -

1.   Most wearable devices have been used for gifting.

2.   Most of the commerce on this segment is online, with 80% of the transactions happening through the digital channel

3.   Majority of the sales happen in the Rs 700- Rs 3000 category of products.

Fitness trackers provide you with a better view of fitness and wellness. Unlike pedometers, physical fitness trackers may help you meet workout goals by adapting to your habits, wirelessly syncing weeks and months of data, and nudging you with quiet vibrating alarms if you have been sitting for too long. Fitness trackers are much more versatile in their monitoring methods and features.

For example, some of them are waterproof, and can help you track activities like swimming.

How can one effectively use a fitness App? This is what I recommend.

1. Keep a daily/ weekly plan

2. As part of the plan keep at least 3 days for outdoor/ vigorous exercise (where possible). This could be walking or spot jogging or even basic stretching

3. If using a tracker, keep the activity to a 30-minute block at the very minimum

4. Measure other outcomes - your weight, how do you feel, how are you sleeping/ resting?

5. Review weekly and modify plan

What also works in the favour of fitness trackers is the possibility of sharing data with a personal trainer and receiving feedback and suggestions on improvement. Many Apps also have a leader board that pushes users to compete with one another by completing certain goals. These achievements can also be shared on social media. In some cases, points are accorded for completion that can be redeemed for gifts or treats.

Mental Health – A beautiful mind

Rahul (name changed) was having a tough time at office. He had worked his way to the top of the tech industry in Bangalore. He was a Senior Vice President at a technology firm and was looking forward to a great time steering the entry of a new technology product in India. But somehow his workload was increasing. What started as a stretch project spanning a few weekends, had consumed him for months? Soon he started dreading the thought of going to office. Even at work his ability to cope with work was reducing, impacting his effectiveness. Soon he was in a cycle, where stress was eating away at his ability to get things done, which contributed to further delays and more stress. Soon panic attacks started occurring in the office. He would sweat profusely and remain tense throughout the day.

Rahul was lucky that he recognised some of the symptoms and sought medical help. He reached out to a counsellor and started treatment immediately. He also took a break from work and focused entirely on his well-being. Slowly, over a period with counselling and medication, Rahul felt better as the incidents of panic attack and their severity started reducing. Before long he was back at a new job, this time with the knowledge that he would have to handle his work better and avoid triggers that might set off the attacks again.

Rahul's case is not an isolated case.

According to a report published by the World Economic Forum in 2014 on the impact of non-communicable diseases on the Indian economy, it is projected that the loss due to poor mental health would be $1.03 trillion before 2030.

Ironically, loss of productivity due to mental health issues is going to cost us more than loss of productivity due to Diabetes and Cancer put together. India it appears is one of the most depressed countries in the world. We have close to 6.7 % of the population that is suffering from some mental illness. And just like Diabetes there is no specific urban/rural divide for this. So, the common perception that people in the villages are not affected by depression is untrue. On the other hand, they may be worse off as there is limited awareness of this and facilities available to address this condition in rural areas. According to a WHO report done by the National Care of Mental Health, suicide rates in India are around 10.7 per lakh of population and victims are mostly below 44 years.

Covid 19 has created an unprecedented scenario where many people are working from home and this has an effect on their mental wellness and health.

People around the world are experiencing a pandemic for the first time in two or three generations. In addition to the rapid spread of the virus, the daily increasing numbers of deaths has triggered anxiety among a lot of people who are worried about their own safety and that of their families. This is even more stressful if any of their loved ones are under quarantine, or worse develop a medical problem.

This is what I recommend as key steps to manage one's mental wellbeing.

- One of the most important things one could do is to cut down on smartphone usage. This can allow us to stay away from the barrage of bad news coming from all over the world, most of which makes us feel helpless as we cannot do anything to help parties involved in the news. This is particularly relevant for children, who out of boredom, might take to excessive usage of the smartphone, which will impact their future psychological development.

- Physical exercise should be undertaken regularly. It can elevate the mood, relieve anxiety and fatigue, and lift a person out of the morose feeling that many are experiencing being stuck in their houses. Any exercise is good but aerobic exercise is especially advised, if possible. Using a treadmill, jogging in the house are some of the options. Physical exercise also acts as an immune booster.

- Yoga and meditation is highly recommended but may be difficult for the uninitiated. Such people can start with simple postures like the Surya Namaskaar etc.

- Breathing exercises can be particularly effective. Even short periods of practice of breathing exercises will have disproportionate benefits. The most effective types are practices including Anulom-Vilom, Bhastrika and Kapalbhati. More patient practitioners can try mindfulness-based meditations. These are widely available on platforms like YouTube etc. It is pertinent to note that, just like with physical exercise, breathing exercises and relief from anxiety also have a positive impact on the immunity. Getting adequate sunlight has well proven benefits too, in this regard.

There are also unexpected benefits from the lockdown. People can now spend more time with their families and can give quality time to their spouses and their children. Catching up on old TV classics like the Ramayana, Mahabharata and Chanakya can be an enjoyable together- time for the family and essential cultural education for the younger generation. Interpersonal interaction with family and friends has its own intrinsic therapeutic potential and catching up with relatives and friends by phone can help in re-establishing old neglected ties and also lead to a sense of oneness in the extended family and the local community that we are all in this together and can get courage and reassurance from each other.

One should also try to make the best use of the time to catch up on long neglected hobbies, practice of the arts and intellectual pursuits like reading, writing and any special projects that we all have planned but never find the time to do. One can enrol oneself in online courses that have been made free by many MOOC (Massive Online Open Courses) providers and upskill themselves and be job-market-ready once the lockdown is over. Gardening is an especially rewarding activity as it promotes both physical and psychological wellbeing.

Some people are also disturbed because of the sudden lack of access to cigarettes and alcohol. This is a valid concern for people used to daily consumption of these substances. Instead of worrying about availability and going out to find these substances, this lockdown can be viewed as a good opportunity to quit these harmful substances. Having some anxiety and sleep disturbances after quitting alcohol is common and can be dealt with by taking mild sedatives (which are prescription drugs and can be obtained only on the advice of a doctor).

More severe withdrawal symptoms can result in withdrawal seizures and delirium which cannot be managed at home and will need the attention of a medical doctor, preferably a psychiatrist.

Despite these measures, if you still experience mental health issues, contact your physician immediately. I did that after the death of my mother and visited a counsellor. Today with the advent of telemedicine, these consultations are anonymous and do not require you to visit a doctor as well.

Seek support from family and friends. I had taken my wife into confidence post my mother's death and she had accompanied me to my counselling session.

Lastly, no matter how bad it may seem, do not attempt self-harm.

In conclusion, poor mental health is a clear and present danger for us in India. Rising expectations and the collapse of work life balance can contribute to this. Work is important but not at the cost of life. But we are creatures of habit and let's look at some key habits that determine our lives.

The usual suspect Part 1 — Sugar

There is something more addictive than cigarettes and alcohol in your diet and you probably don't even know about it. It's **SUGAR**.

Sugar is probably the greatest threat to your health today and you are probably not even aware of it.

I am not talking about the sugar you add to your tea or coffee, but also the sugar that is in processed food like Ketchup, Mayonnaise, and even in healthy food like cornflakes.

Yes, **Cornflakes**,

An article in the Times of India showed the results of some research done on popular Corn Flakes and Muesli brands. The research found that these brands had more than double the sugar prescribed in the corn flakes. According to the European Regulation on Health and Nutritional Claims (ERHNC), "sugar content higher than 12.5 gm per 100 gm is considered to be high'. All variants in the study were found to be exceptionally high in sugar. Not even a single product had printed the sugar content on its packet.

I have personally started experiencing the addiction and control that sugar has on people. Since the lockdown in 2020, to counter the drop in energies while working from home, I had been regularly consuming Cornflakes and Muesli, little realizing that it spiked my sugar levels leading to mood swings, headaches and a general feeling of low spirits. I was consuming a packet of cream biscuits regularly and I gained around 10 kilograms during this time. All this happened while I was still working out and being aware of my consumption.

It took me until the end of June 2020 to figure out what was going on. Since July 2020 I have cut out on most sugar in my diet. Though I have sugar in my coffee and tea but avoid any further sugar in my day. I have swapped out sweets and biscuits with fruit. I know these are early days but I already see an effect on my energy, moods and overall general wellbeing.

Why is sugar so dangerous? Here are some of the reasons from my experience as a doctor and some research that has been publicly released globally.

1. Sugar has no nutritional value. Any sugar that you need can be made by the body from fruits and dairy products. These are naturally occurring sugars and give you fibre, vitamins, and proteins in addition to the sugar.

2. Weight gain is an apparent downside to sugar. Sugar disrupts the Leptin cycle in the body. Leptin is a hormone that regulates the hunger cycles in the body, any disruption in the Leptin cycle can cause weight gain and hunger pangs.

3. Insulin resistance is another reaction to high sugar diets. There is a myth in India that sugar causes diabetes. While sugar does not cause diabetes, but high levels of sugar in the bloodstream leads to insulin production to regulate sugar, and this causes insulin to be less effective over a period of time leading to prediabetes conditions.

4. Lastly sugars are also linked to higher triglycerides level in the body, leading to heart attacks.

5. Switching to Honey or Jaggery as a substitute to sugar has no effect. Like the rules for smoking cessation or alcohol cut out, you need to brutally cut out the sugar, otherwise it will creep back in one spoon at a time.

While it may be challenging to eliminate sugar completely from one's diet, you may try the following measures:

1. Exercise daily

2. Eat only homemade food. That way you can control the amount of sugar you are adding to the food. But this is not a license to make homemade mithai loaded with sugar

3. Check the added sugar quantity before buying anything from the market. Make it a rule of thumb that added sugar should not be more than 10 % of the ingredients. But best would be to avoid products with any added sugar

4. Load your diet with fruits and vegetables. Some fruits like Bananas and Chickoo are loaded with sugar, but at the same time these are natural sugars and are less harmful but if possible avoid fruits with high sugar content.

Like the monitoring of diet and Vitamin D Levels, sugar intake also needs to be monitored. One of the ways of doing this is to set a quota for sugar consumption every week. Make only that much sugar available and the rest of it can be hidden away or made difficult to access. This way you can see your consumption every day. One of the things my wife did to stem my midnight biscuit eating habits, was to hide biscuits beneath a heap of other grocery items, making it difficult for me to reach. Now let's look at another habit forming ingredient salt.

The usual suspect Part 2 – Salt

While we have discussed the dangers of sugar, let us now look at another usual suspect that hides in plain sight - Salt. Salt is a very important source of Sodium for our body, and Sodium is very important for the transmission of messages for our nervous system. Sodium, along with Potassium, are important channel drivers in our body, and almost every message, or neural impulse that passes between the various nodes in our body is through the interactions between Sodium and Potassium. So how is salt suddenly so dangerous?

According to research, it is estimated that an average Indian has anywhere between 2500, to 4000, milligrams of Sodium per day. That translates to almost 10 to 12 grams of salt.

Salt, also naturally occurs in many food items like vegetables and fruit, as well as grains. But the most important source of salt for us is added salt that is put in our daily food. But when the meal includes pre-processed foods, like chips or savoury snacks, our salt levels can increase by three times. In turn, this can cause Sodium levels to rise, resulting in water retention, aggravating high blood pressure, diabetes and kidney disease.

(Patients suffering from these ailments are expected to consume much lesser quantity of Sodium per day, below even the 2000 milligrams of Sodium per day).

If you don't suffer from any of these ailments, increased salt intake over time can lead to spiking in blood pressure levels and weight gain due to water retention.

Processed food can also mask the true flavour of ingredients by adding more salt and spices, with a view to make it tasty and preserve it for longer. Even simple foods like soup powders, have a high degree of salt and a high degree of Sodium added to them.

If you very carefully look at the package of a processed food like say salted peanuts, or masala peanuts, you will see the calorific content and other nutrition content of the food item. There will be a mention of either Sodium or salt, which is added as a natural preservative. Leading brands may also mention if the Sodium levels in the product correspond to the amount of Sodium required for one meal in a day. Preservatives like 211 are very common in processed food, this preservative is Sodium Benzoate and is common in most foods like sauce and spread. This means, if the packet of soup has adequate Sodium for one meal, you are not expected to complement the soup with other items like bread, which may add more Sodium for that meal.

So what can you do to reduce your salt intake?

First and foremost, try to have more home cooked meals. Initially add slightly less salt than what you are used to. Over time, a gradual reduction in salt will help our taste buds adjust better, than a radical reduction in salt levels.

Add other spices, such as pepper or cardamom that can flavour your food well, thereby reducing reliance on salt.

In case you are unable to cook at home and rely on packaged food, check the labels for salt content. Try having substitutes for popular snacks. Unsalted peanuts or boiled peanuts can be a substitute for masala peanuts. If you have any canned food or canned vegetables or fruit, make sure you wash them very well, to remove salt.

In case you dine out, try mentioning to the restaurant that you need a low salt meal.

Alcohol – no more shots please

Alcoholism has many negative connotations in India. Not only is it considered an unfavourable practice but also one which is banned on religious days. Despite the social and religious taboos, alcohol is being consumed by 25-50 % of men in most regions of the country.

Though most of the recent references to alcohol are in the urban areas, where growing western lifestyle is seeing young men and women consuming beverages laden with alcohol, the severe socio-economic implications of this practice are in the rural hinterlands.

My interest in the subject started one day during a visit to Kerala. I was there to attend a conference and to my amazement, I found out that all wine shops were closed in Kerala on the first day of the month. This was because all salaries were given on the first day of the month and most men would take that money directly to the liquor shop rather than the bank or the house.

In fact, an average male in Kerala consumes 8 litres of alcohol - double the country average for India. Some states in the country like Mizoram, Manipur and Gujrat have banned the consumption of alcohol. Many other states have revised age limits for alcohol consumption.

Alcohol leads to some health implications, which in turn lead to economic implications for the affected families. The most common condition associated with alcohol is cirrhosis of the liver. Other complications include- Diabetes Mellitus, Cancer, Coronary heart Disease, poisoning and epilepsy.

But the most important complication resulting from this is the addictive nature of alcohol consumption which often leads to repeat purchase and is currently driving the growth of the Industry. In rural India, the use of alcohol leads to loss of pay. Most workers in these areas are working on daily wages and the inability to work due to intoxication results in loss of pay.

To add to this is the complex problem of not having Government health insurance coverage, which leads to workers and their families taking loans from money lenders, which finally leads to their perdition.

Alcohol education has been successfully used in many countries as a tool to help with de-addiction. Government channels like All India Radio run programs in various languages focusing on the challenges with Alcohol and its implications. Also many NGOs have started working with women and educating them on dealing with alcoholic husbands and safeguarding themselves from the domestic violence that can follow. Interestingly many tea and coffee estate owners in South India now hand over the monthly salaries of the workers to their wives to stop these men from wasting salaries on Alcohol.

But in cities alcohol has a different connotation, especially in the context of Diabetes.

We often hear that diabetics need to control their diet and avoid sugar. But can they consume alcohol?

The most important rule is to keep alcohol consumption moderate. Studies have shown that moderate alcohol consumption may have positive health effects like raising HDL (good) cholesterol and lowering the risk of cardiovascular disease. Other studies suggest that moderate alcohol consumption may even reduce risk of type 2 diabetes. The American Heart Association defines moderate alcohol consumption as 1 drink a day for women and 2 drinks a day for men. For reference, a single drink is measured as a 12 oz. beer, a 5 oz. glass of wine, or 1 ½ oz. of distilled spirits i.e. vodka, whisky, gin etc.

However, excessive alcohol consumption or binge drinking, in which a person consumes more than 5 drinks in a two-hour span of time for men and 4 for women, can increase the risk of heart disease, type 2 diabetes, and metabolic syndrome. Alcohol in excess can further increase your weight which can lead to insulin resistance making glucose control more challenging.

A person living with type 2 diabetes is free to consume alcohol if desired, however, additional safety measures should be taken. Some alcoholic beverages are better than others for type 2 diabetics and other tips should be followed in order to stay safe. The American Diabetes Association recommends that individuals living with diabetes should be able to recognize and manage delayed hypoglycaemia (low blood sugar) when drinking alcohol especially if these individuals use insulin or other medications that can cause blood sugar levels to drop. Since alcohol consumption can result in increased insulin production which can lower blood sugar levels, education is vital for safety.

What you shouldn't drink

Diabetics should avoid sugary drinks mixed with processed juices, added sugars and artificial syrups which can add high doses of processed sugars. Such beverages can cause blood glucose spikes and weight gain if consumed in excess.

What you should drink

Alcoholic beverages like wine, champagne or distilled alcohol mixed with seltzer water or club soda are better options for diabetics. So instead of ordering that vodka cranberry, try a vodka with club soda with a squeeze of lime.

Drink with food

Should you decide to consume alcohol occasionally, never drink on an empty stomach. Have your drink with a meal or eat right before you drink to reduce the risk of hypoglycaemia. Your food should include carbohydrates so that some glucose will be in your system when you drink, lowering your risk of hypoglycaemia. Feel free to consume as many carbohydrates as you need while drinking and never replace food with alcohol or count alcohol as part of your daily intake of carbohydrates.

If you are taking insulin or other medications that can lower blood sugar, prepare ahead of time and have some snacks on hand. Meals can have a delayed reaction in the body so snacks can come in handy. This can come in the form of a piece of whole grain toast, an apple or a bowl of oats with berries. These foods have also shown to help type 2 diabetics manage blood glucose and weight.

Drink with water

If you think you might drink more than 1 or 2 alcoholic beverages in a single night, drink a glass water or club soda in between each drink. The more hydrated you are; the less alcohol you will drink.

Keep your medical records handy

Keeping your medical records handy at all times is ideal. In case of a medical emergency health professionals will know about your condition. However, if you prefer not to keep the records with you, at least inform a family member on your whereabouts.

Monitor blood sugar

In the end, the only way to know what works for you is to monitor your blood sugar more often while drinking alcohol. Even 24 hours after drinking, alcohol can cause a drop in blood sugar.

So, safety first and bottoms up later.

Smoking is just another day in paradise

A few months ago, I was a part of an expert panel that was doing an audit of the health policies of an organisation. The audit is called Healthy Workplace Audit and it has various parameters that are assessed right from flexible work timings to having cafeterias and canteens that serve healthy food.

The one thing that struck me about the audit was the emphasis it placed on smoking cessation and creating a smoke free workplace. Ever since the government of India has passed the bill to eliminate smoking in public spaces, I see a lot of effort being put in by the government and private organisation to reduce smoking.

Smoking is not a few phenomenon in the country. There is evidence of Bhang and Cannabis consumption for almost 2000 years. It is even prescribed in ancient texts as a medicinal practice to manage pain and neurological disorders. Most recently Hookah has been used by both the royalty as well as the common people.

But tobacco also accounts for almost 10 million deaths in the country. Add to it the impact it has on the cardiovascular system and respiratory system, would make it a very lethal habit to cultivate. Cigarettes for example contain more than 7000 chemicals out of which more than 250 are harmful and more than 60 are carcinogenic. Non Communicable diseases also continue to be boosted by the habit of chewing and smoking tobacco. Cigarettes also contain another addictive substance- Sugar as one of the ingredients, it might as well be that the sugar is causing the addiction and not the nicotine.

While India has implemented many laws including Cigarettes and Other Tobacco Products Act (COTPA) with the creation of a National Tobacco Control Programme (NTCP) in 2007, the reason for the continued use of tobacco can be attributed to the economics of it.

Today the tobacco industry caters to almost 120 million customers in India. The vast majority of tobacco is grown in Karnataka, Andhra Pradesh, and Gujrat. Almost 50% of the tobacco consumed in India is the chewable type used in Gutka, Khaini and Zarda. Almost 30% as bidis and only about 20% as cigarettes.

The revenue for the government from the sale of tobacco products is around Rs 43,000 crores.

While it is complex to understand how one can reduce consumption while balancing the potential loss in revenue, from a medical standpoint, below are some suggestions to help smokers reduce their consumption.

1.   Treat smoking or chewing of tobacco as addiction. If you think you are addicted, please enter therapy just like how we would expect people with drug addiction to undergo therapy.

2.   Focus on nutrition and health. One of the reasons why tobacco consumption is very popular, is because many people do not receive adequate nutrition. Tobacco consumption quells hunger and that's the sole reason why it should be tackled. So long working hours and compensating for nutrition is often supplemented with tobacco.

3.   Create smoking zones and tobacco consumption zones all over cities to ensure that the concentration of efforts to manage the communication and addiction can be well coordinated. Ban all consumption outside of these zones.

An average Indian urban smoker, smokes about 6.8 Cigarettes a day and on an average spends close to INR 1200 per month on cigarettes. That's a lot of money on something that adds no nutritional value and instead causes you more harm. A casual cigarette or Cigar is different but processed cigarettes have many ingredients that are addictive, including sugar and research believes that sugar adds to the addictive nature of the product. So this is what I want you to do, each time you feel like smoking take that money equivalent and put it in an envelope or a piggy bank. At the end of the month count that money. You will see substantial savings. That's the best way to beat the habit, economically. Now let's look at some good lifestyle changes that you can adopt.

Ayurveda – medicine from the Gods

China today dominates the herbal medicine market. One of the reasons for that is branding.

In many ways the natural leader in that market should have been India. Unfortunately, we as a nation have missed that bus in the 1950-70's. Ayurveda, our core herbal offering to the world, lay mired in home enterprises which never concentrated on branding. Most remedies were dispensed as powders, given in unmarked sachets, with little or no standardization on packaging or consumer literature that one sees with other allopathic offerings.

In that gap, China catapulted itself in the global space. Today Chinese traditional medicine popularised by the Kung- Fu movies has travelled far more than the Indian science of Ayurveda. According to a report by Global Industry Analysts, the market is estimated to be $ 120 Billion by 2025. The rate of growth of the market is around 9 %. The largest market for these therapies remains Europe while Asia Pacific as a market is the fastest growing.

Herbal therapies have received a shot in the arm from the adoption of the cGMP (Good Manufacturing Practices) by most of these firms as prescribed by the FDA. Also there is a growing feeling within the patient community to adopt herbal medicines from a prevention and diet supplement point of view.

The other trend in this space is a shift by many manufacturers from single ingredient formulation to a multi ingredient formulation with a focus on the outcomes. This shift from source to outcome is also leading to a spurt in the growth of herbal medicines.

With China slated to dominate this market, what can Indian manufacturers do?

For one they can take a cue from Dabur and Himalaya and focus on branding their products. Dabur, for example, is one of the leading Indian Ayurveda brands and continues to lead the charge on getting India the rightful place in the Global Herbal market.

Secondly many firms might have to adopt the cGMP practices as laid down by the FDA. This will lead to opening up of many markets especially in Europe and America.

Thirdly firms need to spend time on patient education, letting both Indian and global consumers know the benefits of using Ayurveda. I do feel that many young Indians associate Ayurveda with the older vision of India and do not want to adopt it. During a recent trip to a Naattu Marandu (Traditional Ayurveda) Shop in Chennai I saw that most customers were in the age group of 50 plus. As a matter of fact, many in my peer group found it funny that I was buying traditional medicine despite being trained in Allopathy.

How can you adopt

1. Ayurveda is a great alternative when it comes to dealing with Lifestyle and chronic conditions

2. Find a good vaid (Ayurvedic doctor). There are many Ayurveda centres in India, those from Kottakal in Kerala are very famous, please look for those centers. Also Patanjali has chikitshalay's associated with them, a simple google search will help you there.

3. Change your life style as per the guidance of the vaid, remember Ayurveda does not help in acute condition, please look for Ayurveda as ways and means to change your lifestyle

Today Ayurveda is looked at as a reminder of the old India. It is time to change that. We can look at our traditional diet and Ayurveda and adopt them as citizens of the new India.

Let's now look at Yoga and how it can promote, health and happiness.

The Magic of Yoga

Yoga was first introduced to the modern world after Swami Vivekananda travelled and spoke at the Parliament of World Religions which was held in Chicago in 1893. Not only did he introduce Yoga to the west, it also led to re-invigoration of the practice of Yoga in India. Since then numerous Indian and Western health experts have come forward talking about the benefits of Yoga. Recently the International Day of Yoga' was celebrated across the world with participants from very diverse countries like Tunisia, Venezuela and New Zealand.

Yoga predates the Vedic period and makes its first appearance in the Rig Veda. Historically the earliest records of yoga were found in the 5th and 6th century BCE. Some records of Yoga were also found in the Katha Upanishad.

Greek historians travelling with Alexander the Great have recorded encounters with Yogis, who had developed a sense of aloofness and were seen in various postures, some sitting and some standing and they refused to meet the Greek visitors. Yoga has references in the Buddhist Pali Canons and the Bhagwat Gita.

The practice of Yoga developed across the ages, imparting physical, mental and spiritual health to its practitioners. These are some key benefits that have helped me-

- Circulatory system improvement- Yoga has known to have remarkable benefits to long time users to the musculoskeletal system. Practicing Yoga leads to the increase in the GABA levels that helps control moods and reduce anxiety. The breathing exercises as part of yoga lead to improved cardiac rehabilitation improves asthma, and in some cases known to lower the blood pressure. When I was having some breathing issues mostly due to allergy, a 20-minute Yoga session went a long way in improving the circulation and breathing.

- Lower back rehabilitation- Most of us with sedentary work lifestyle have suffered from back pain at some point in our lives. It is not uncommon to see a 20-year-old with back problems. Yoga has an effect on the skeletal system and is known to relieve the stress in the lower back. Research done by the Boston University school of medicine shows that Yoga combined with rehabilitation for lower back led to reduction of pain for 1/3 rd of the volunteer group, as opposed to only 5 % of the control group that did not combine Yoga with their post-operative care. The percentage drop for those taking pain medication also reduced by almost 80% for the volunteer group. I have used Yoga to reduce any stress on the back and to reduce back pain. In an earlier piece I wrote about how you can improve your health while in office. I can easily add a few Yogic exercises to it and the benefits would double.

- For Sports- Yoga has been effective in reducing sports injuries and helping sportsmen recover and gain overall fitness. It has prolonged the playing career of many sportsmen including footballer Ryan Giggs who played for Manchester United and Wales beyond the age of 40. Yoga gives internal strength to the muscles and the skeletal system. It helps increase the blood supply to the muscles. During professional sports or during training, the tightening of muscles reduces the blood supply and this increases the chances of injury

Everyday new benefits of Yoga are discovered, and they are then empirically proven in research. In 2014 the UN passed a resolution to celebrate June 21st as the International Day for Yoga or IDY.

So how can you get started with Yoga

1. Read up on Yoga – Being Indians most of us are aware of Yoga, having seen or heard of some family friend or relative practicing it. Now, thanks to the Government propagating the International Day for Yoga, there is even greater awareness. To understand what Yoga can do for you, I suggest you start by reading on the Internet. If you would like to seek specific guidance relating to an ailment, then its best to reach out to a yoga teacher and ask for a customized routine.

2. Set realistic expectations – While doing research on Yoga one comes across several schools of thought. Pick a branch of Yoga whose philosophy you are comfortable with. For example, I don't look at Yoga as a tool to lose weight or cure myself of an ailment. To me, Yoga is for improving flexibility and feeling good. I don't seek perfection (such as getting a posture right or holding the breath for exactly 60 seconds etc). My expectations therefore are set accordingly. Yoga may not be a substitute for a high intensity workout that may help you lose 3 Kgs a month. But if you are looking for better health (mental and physical) over a 12-24 month period or longer, Yoga can help.

3. Don't wait for a good day or time to start – Unlike other forms of exercise that may require lots of energy, and therefore get restricted to either early mornings or late evenings, Yoga can be done pretty much any time of the day, as long as you give at least an hour's gap post eating food. Further, you don't need a specific outfit or props to get started with Yoga.

4. Last but not the least, like every Indian practice, Yoga needs a guru. Try to find a Yoga guru in your area or someone who takes online classes. A guru will guide you correctly and help you master the practices associated with yoga.

But Yoga is not all movement, it is also nutrition and medication. Let's discuss a few hacks that you can learn from Yoga.

Five simple hacks from yoga

Below are my observations on how yoga and Ayurveda prescribe nutrition and what we can learn from that.

I have been watching my nutrition for a while. I've read numerous books, tracked my meals on an App for a year and visited a few nutritionists to figure out portion sizes, calories and supplements. One person (who could have made a great psychologist) even told me that I should visualize happiness whenever I saw a raw vegetable and think of something evil and disgusting every time, I came in the vicinity of anything fried or sweet.

After going on crash diets and then binge eating, it came to a point where I just gave up and continued eating what I felt like eating. For example, if I avoided sugar for a week, I would feel like having a toffee or small bar of chocolate and I would give in. This of course made me feel guilty of being unable to cultivate good eating habits. And it was not easy considering my family eat whatever they want to – including sweets and fried snacks almost daily alongside healthy food- and continue to stay healthy. My father has told me never to skimp on food. "It's a basic need, just like clothing and shelter. One that we all earn money for", he would say.

Imagine my surprise, when I read the same lines in a book on Yoga that my friend lent me. I was reading a chapter on obesity and how to cure oneself of it, when I read the line. "Don't compromise on food. Eat nutritious food and include indulgences too – as many times as the body wants." The rest of the chapter challenged my way of thinking towards food and diets in general. I tried whatever was suggested for a couple of days and felt physical and mentally happier. Some of these measures are listed below.

1. On Portion sizes – As per yogic tradition, portion sizes are dependent on individual body needs. There is no one-size-fits-all. Your portion size is whatever quantity of food is required to make you feel full. If that means 4 chapatis for dinner, so be it. I have relied on several western methods to calculate portion sizes and found it impractical to my situation. For example, one version says a person should eat 2 palm sized portions of carbohydrates, 2 fist full of proteins, a thumb sized portion of fats, and two portions of greens/ vegetables/ fruits, as large as your hands can make an open bowl shape when joined together. The challenge with Indian food is that most dishes usually combine one or more food groups. For example – what does a Dal with vegetables amount to? Protein or carbs or greens? Should I then have 2 bowlfuls of dal but only 1 chapati? In contrast, the yogic advice on portion sizes was practical. On most days I feel full with 2 chapatis, 2-3 helpings of subzi. I have stuck to following that pattern for a while now and not observed any adverse reactions.

2. On counting calories – While most of us know that fried and sweet food isn't healthy, what we don't know is that the body inherently cannot take in more than a certain amount of these foods. That's why most people tend to feel sick after overdosing on chips or sweets. For those of us who cannot restrain ourselves from overdosing, Yoga suggests external intervention from experts as this could indicate a deeper problem – depression, gut related issues etc. But for those of us who don't eat sweets

or fried food regularly, indulgences, even fairly regular ones, are ok. Yoga says that a healthy body indicates its need for certain foods that it has been deprived of. Cravings for sweets and fried foods falls in the same category. So if you have gone without sugar for a week, you will be tempted to eat a bar of chocolate to compensate for it. I generally avoid drinking any beverage because of the sugar added in. But this time, I tried drinking a glass of plain milk with a spoonful of sugar for a week. I had no cravings for anything remotely sugar. Eventually I discontinued the practice because I felt milk was making me feel full and interfered with my regular meals. So these days, if I crave sugar, I have a spoonful of it or grab a couple of toffees and get one with life.

3. On water – While we are aware that one needs 8 glasses of water or roughly 2 litres, it is difficult to monitor this strictly. It's no secret that we drink less water during colder weather and more in summers. But regulating water intake is necessary for proper functioning of our organs. Yoga suggests that we drink water after meals and in between meals to keep hunger at bay. Before meals, warm water or soups/ rasam can be taken to reduce hunger, especially by those looking to lose weight. I have personally tried this for several years now, and my food intake has been reduced by 30% due to the increased water intake. In the West too, the benefits of water are recognized and the gallon challenge is testimony to that.

4. On eating multiple meals – for the last 5-6 years I have seen Indian nutritionists and fitness professionals insisting on eating 6-8 small meals throughout the day. While this works for many people, for me the mere thought of constantly chomping on something every 2 hours is painful. I have always eaten 3-4 square meals and find it impossible to eat anything else, as

that in turn affects my other meals. The book I was reading indicated that most Yogis survive on 2 full meals and eat them by 10:00 am and 5:00 pm, giving the body ample time to digest them. If they felt hungry in between, they just drank water, buttermilk or hot soup. Most food takes anywhere between 3-4 hours to digest. Eating every 2 hours may not give enough digestion time. So for those who fret because they are unable to eat 6-8 meals, there is nothing wrong in eating 3-4 square meals.

5. On feeling full – Knowing when to stop is the key to developing good food habits. Yoga says one must listen for cues/ signals from the brain to tell you when you are full. I found this to be the most difficult aspect of getting my eating act right. Most of us tend to not focus on food. I for one, love to read a book while eating (to escape feeling depressed about how tiny my portions are). My older daughter needs to be told a story while being fed. My wife usually checks his mails or takes a call while dining. Net result – the brain is unable to send you signals pertaining to hunger because it's sending you signals on something else. Like, assimilating what happens in the story next or planning how to respond to a question asked during an office call. Even if it sends us cues on food, we miss them because of our lack of focus. To help me understand when I felt full, I tried this experiment. The results shocked me. I had one chapati with subzi and then waited for 3-4 minutes. Surprisingly, I felt full. This was half my meal. I waited longer to see if I hadn't been misled. But no, I didn't feel hungry any more. Trying this over a week though, I realized the stomach was getting full at 1.5 chapatis and 2 helpings of subzi. So the half chapatti and one more cup of subzi I had been regularly eating had been extra – amounting to overeating of some sort.

Instead of following complicated eating patterns, if I had just listened to my stomach, I would know when to stop eating and be able to manage my weight better.

Trying some of these methods worked for me and made me feel positive about my eating habits. They may or may not work for all. But there's no harm in trying them out, as they don't cost anything and are unlikely to do any bodily harm (unless you suffer from an existing health condition). Again, Yoga is best practiced under a guru. While Yoga and Ayurveda keep you fit, there is the question of nutrition. Let's see how to track that.

Cornflakes, breakfast of champions?

India is facing an obesity epidemic. Currently an estimated 30 million people in India currently would fall under the obese category.

With this market in place, many organizations have decided to make a play to help us lose weight and fight the obesity epidemic. There are gyms, specialty clinics, fitness diets and portions.

The latest entrant in this market is Cornflakes. The firm has been trying to make inroads into India for a long time. Their initial entry did not work well as a breakfast alternative. The point is that Indians unlike the westerners like hot breakfast. Cornflakes on the other hand is recommended to be consumed with cold milk and not hot milk.

After years of trying to fight that battle in India, the brand came to the position that we could have it anyway we wanted either with hot milk or cold milk. But this positioning was for the children and young adults. In addition, they tried positioning it as a supplement having essential minerals like Iron and other micro nutrients that boosted academic performance.

Lately cornflakes have been positioned as a panacea for all those who want to lose weight. Especially targeting women who are generally more weight conscious. But is Cornflakes good for us?

In the earlier chapter I referred to the 2009 article in Times of India showed the results of some research done on popular Corn Flakes and Muesli brands.

According to an article in the public media, not only are cornflakes unhealthy for breakfast, they should be totally avoided by anyone trying to lose weight. A box of cornflakes contains the following- Corn, Sugar, Malt, Corn Syrup high on Fructose. These ingredients especially the Corn syrup contain High Glycaemic Index(GI) Carbohydrates. What a high GI carbohydrate does is raise the level of sugar rapidly in the blood stream. This causes the brain to direct the pancreas to release insulin. The release of insulin automatically decreases the sugar level. This creates a situation where the body is suddenly without sugar and feels lazy and lifeless. Most of us would have experienced that situation after a white rice or a white bread meal. Brain then sends an automatic signal to the body to resume eating as a false sense of starvation leads to further eating. As a matter of fact, an adult size portion of cornflakes consists of almost 350 calories. This means it has high carbohydrates and less proteins, making it a very dangerous meal for diabetics and those in the pre-diabetes phase.

So technically a Corn Flakes diet cannot help one in losing weight and would not lead to children having a balanced diet as breakfast just before school.

In another report it is stated that the Iron levels in cornflakes is much lower than the prescribed levels. Referring again the article in Times of India and I quote" The study also found that compared to the published iron content on the packaging of 23.3 mg per 100 gm, the results showed that corn flakes with real banana and mango, contained only 8.7 mg to 12.3 mg of iron per 100 gm."

In addition, India has around 50 Million diabetics and also has the famous belly gene which already causes obesity related complications especially among the upper strata of society.

In conclusion through Corn Flakes is a tasty meal we probably should not use it as an alternative to either a balanced diet or exercise. A good breakfast would still be Fruits and Vegetables followed by a traditional Indian fare like Idly or Upma.

Let's look at the humble Idly in the next chapter and get some insights into how we have the breakfast of champions.

Idli more than cornflakes can make your day

According to a breakfast survey done at 4 major metros in 2013 in India, Idli-sambar came out on tops as the most nutritious breakfast. This combination won over modern additions like bread and Cornflakes. A mix of rice and urad dal (White Lentil), the Idli is an ideal mix of protein, fat and carbohydrates with the Sambar providing vitamins and minerals.

Needless to say Chennai came out tops as the city where almost 60 % of those surveyed consumed this breakfast. Interestingly most of the nation did not consume breakfast or did not consume enough of it.

The research was sponsored by Kellogg's who have been trying for last 20 years to get some foothold in the Indian breakfast table as descried in the previous chapter.

Interestingly the late Tamilnadu chief Minister Dr. Jayalalitha inaugurated a corporation run restaurant in 2013 which would serve Idli-Sambar for Rs 10. These outlets are called Amma Unavagam or Amma Canteen and 13 such outlets were opened in February 2013 and there were plans to open 100 more in the year. In 2020 there are more than 500 outlets that are serving more than 11 lakhs people daily for free, due to the pandemic and subsequent lockdown. The state governments of Karnataka and Rajasthan had launched Indira Canteens and Annapurna Rasoi respectively inspired by the Amma Canteens.

Nutrition Facts

Serving Size	1 piece
	Per serve
Energy	**169 kj**
	40 kcal
Fat	**0.19g**
Saturated Fat	0.037g
Monounsaturated Fat	0.035g
Polyunsaturated Fat	0.043g
Carbohydrates	**7.89g**
Sugar	0.22g
Fibre	1.5g
Protein	**1.91g**
Sodium	207mg
Cholesterol	0mg
Potassium	63mg

Diagram 15 Nutritional content of idli shows it has the right balance between protein and carbohydrates

The History of Idli

Historically Idli was first mentioned by the Kannada historian and King Someshwara III in 1170 AD. It seems to have been influenced by the Indonesian style of steam cooking. But there are multiple theories about the origins of Idli.

A precursor of the modern Idli is mentioned in several ancient Indian works. *Vaddaradhane*, a 920 CE Kannada language work by Shivakotiacharya mentions "iddalige", prepared only from a black gram batter.

Chavundaraya II, the author of the earliest available Kannada encyclopedia, *Lokopakara* (c. 1025 CE), describes the preparation of this food by soaking black gram in buttermilk, ground to a fine paste, and mixed with the clear water of curd and spices. The Western Chalukya king and scholar Someshwara III, reigning in the area now called Karnataka, included an idli recipe in his encyclopedia, *Manasollasa* (1130 CE).

This Sanskrit-language work describes the food as *iḍḍarikā*. In Karnataka, the Idli in 1235 CE is described as being 'light, like coins of high value', which is not suggestive of a rice base. The food prepared using this recipe is now called *uddina idli* in Karnataka.

But in a further twist there are claims that Idli originated from Indonesia. The vegetarian cooks of the Hindu kings of Indonesia were the ones who invented the Idli and then it found its way to India. There are also theories that Idli was introduced to south India from Saurashtra through the businessmen there.

Whatever the origins, Idli has the ability to become the breakfast of India. And here are my reasons

1. Good for Kids- High in Carbohydrates and Proteins- That means Idli is good for children. It's an excellent breakfast for kids and knowing the extent of the malnutrition issues in the country, this would be a good way to address them. Also the Amma Canteens are a good step in the right direction and they should be replicated across the country

2. For the senior citizens- Malnutrition is an issue that extends across both ends of the spectrum, while we can cover the children, I think Idli would help us cover the senior citizens as well.

3. Healthy start to the day- It is a good start to the day, easy to digest and made totally with local incidents. With the right appliance like a wet grinder the batter can be made at home.

4. Idli can also be made with Millets, the low cost variant that even the Niti Ayog is espousing as a cure for India's long term food problems.

I would like to encourage all of you to start looking at local foods like the Idli to make a great start to the day as well as fulfil the nutritional requirements of the entire family. Here Idli is just an example. Please go back to your elders, grandparents and grand aunts and check with them what did they eat traditionally? Are there traditional foods that they were consuming all these years? Please stick to those.

I see a lot of young people take to Keto diets or go gluten free and even indulge in some exotic cereal like Quinoa. I am not a dietician and don't know how to respond to that but common sense tells me if that if these diets didn't exist in India previously, can they actually be good for us?

Think local. One of the biggest lessons I learn from watching Gordon Ramsey Kitchen Nightmares was to look at local produce and procure locally. See what grows in your regions and consume that only. Get vocal for local for food as well as this only is good for taste but also boosts your immune system. Let discuss more in the next chapter.

Boost your immunity for good health

Immunity is the ability of the body to resist the attack of pathogens, or to fight against the infection which is caused due to unwanted biological invasion. It is an indication of the tolerance level of the host to strike back against the infection, reacting by the action of specific antibodies.

For the immune system to function well, it requires balance and harmony. However, there are times when this system fails – a germ invades successfully, some biological changes happen and make us sick. Many questions arise in these cases: Whether there are any ways to intervene in this process and make our system stronger? Any helpful dietary changes? Any supplements required?

Well the answer to all of these questions is to adopt a healthy living to boost immunity. The most important formula for a healthy immune system is

BALANCED DIET + EXERCISE =HEALTHY IMMUNE SYSTEM

Some key points to remember are

- Pick a diet rich in vegetables, fruits, low in saturated fat

- Maintaining healthy weight, this can be measured by BMI

- Exercising regularly – I would recommend 150 minutes of workout per week

- Manage and regulate blood pressure, there are good home BP monitors available, very important to monitor your BP- As discussed earlier I use an Omron BP Monitor similar monitors are available

- Moderate smoking and drinking alcohol, if you can refrain even better

- Get adequate sleep, at least 8 hours of sleep is recommended by the WHO

- Regular medical screening tests based on age group and risk category.

In addition to these, Vitamins play an important role in boosting immunity, here are some key Vitamins

Vitamin	Role	Sources
C	**Biggest immunity booster. Daily intake is essential as our body does not produce or store it.**	**Citrus, Berries, Spinach, Broccoli**
B6	**Pivotal role in catalysing the biochemical reaction in the immune system.**	**Green vegetables, Chicken, ChickPeas**
E	**Powerful antioxidant – Helps in fighting off infection.**	**Nuts, Seeds, Spinach**

Diagram 16 List of the three top vitamins or boosting immunity. This is in addition to Vitamin D and Vitamin B12 that we have already discussed

Avoid supplements

Sometimes we do end up taking prescribed supplements specially to boost immunity during sickness. But it is best not to make them a habit and to absorb nutrients through natural sources.

So things to remember so far...

1. Immunity is important for good health

2. Immunity can be boosted by a combination of diet and exercise

3. Vitamins are key for boosting immunity

4. Avoid supplements, the best way to gain nutrition is from natural sources

But another key component is keeping the stomach healthy so that it can absorb all these nutrients. Let's see how we can do that.

The key to your lifestyle is through your stomach

Modern lifestyles, improper dietary habits and eating junk food can place a huge strain on the digestive system. Problems with digestion can affect every other part of your body and bring down your quality of life. As the English author Samuel Johnson said, "He who does not mind his belly, will hardly mind anything else." Caring for your digestion is not difficult. Here are a few simple ways to do it.

Eat a high fiber diet

Eating lots of vegetables, fruits and grains that are rich in fiber will enable food to move smoothly through the digestive system and reduce the strain on it. This also helps to prevent Irritable Bowel Syndrome and Haemorrhoids.

Eat the right balance of fiber

Insoluble fiber or roughage cannot be digested by the system and so it adds bulk to the stools, making a bowel movement easier. Soluble fiber absorbs excess water and keeps the stools from becoming too liquid. A balance of both types of fiber is important.

Ensure probiotic intake

Not all bacteria are bad. Probiotics are a type of healthy bacteria that helps to support the digestive process, strengthen the immune system and accelerates the natural breakdown of food by the body.

Drink lots of water

Staying hydrated by drinking enough water has all kinds of health benefits, including on the digestive system. Water acts as a lubricant, enabling the smooth digestion of food and elimination of waste from the body.

Keep regular mealtimes

Eating your breakfast, lunch and dinner at as near as possible at the same time every day means that your body is provided nourishment at the right interval thereby preventing the digestion from being overloaded by sudden large food intakes and also by not allowing the stomach to remain empty for long periods, which results in acidity and other problems.

Get enough exercise

Exercise is usually looked at as a way to lose weight and not being overweight is good for overall health. More than this, exercise supports the digestive system and the movement of the body keeps pushing food through the digestive system, which enables good bowel movements and prevents constipation.

Reduce stress

Mental stress and anxiety place a great strain on the digestive system and prevent it from functioning properly. It can cause all kinds of digestion-related medical conditions including the development of ulcers in the stomach. Make stress-reducing activities like Yoga a part of your daily schedule.

Avoid questionable habits

Smoking, excessive consumption of alcohol and tea or coffee all interfere with the smooth functioning of the digestion. If the habits cannot be totally removed from your life, then very moderate consumption is the next best step. In any case avoid added sugar.

While nutrition is the key to health, on the other end of the spectrum there is malnutrition both with children and adults. Now let's look at that as well.

No food for thought, malnutrition is a real problem

In the August of 2020, cases in India for Covid19 had crossed the 2 million mark. While the fatality remained low as a percentage at 2.7%, the growth in cases was on an upward trend. One of the key aspects that Covid19 has exposed is our broken healthcare system.

Food and diet is one of the key parameters that make or break our health. While the world focuses on obesity, there is a silent killer in our midst. Obesity is one aspect that is heavily covered in media in India. There are numerous reports on how the 'Fight against Fat' is the paradigm shift in Indian public health policy. Obesity has been linked to heart diseases, diabetes and hypertension. And the information is all correct.

But I believe in a country of a billion people plus a problem affecting 50-60 million people is hardly the real story. Let's take the case of diabetes for example, the situation today affects about 50 million people with another 30-40 million undetected cases.

But the silent killer is Malnutrition.

India's greatest challenge is malnutrition.

So all those basic biology classes on balanced diet are the need of the hour for India. This has become more apparent in Covid19, as the foundational health of the individual has implications on his or her recovery rate.

According to a report by the UN and the World Bank, India is ranked second in the number of children suffering from malnutrition. The other country ahead of us is Bangladesh. Almost 47 % of the children in India are affected by this condition.

Another alarming statistic is that India has about 150 million children contributing almost 18 % of the population. Also four children die every minute from preventable diseases like Diarrhoea, Measles and Typhoid which are usually more severe due to the prevalent malnutrition.

The icing on the cake is the 2019 Global Hunger Index (GHI) where India is ranked 102 out of 117 countries. Some of the other countries on the list are very small and poorer than us, but still have shown improvement. Sri Lanka for example has an index score of 14, while India lands an alarming 23.7. Even Niger has a score of 23.

But Media and industry continue to focus on obesity. The reasons are very simple. The obese population are also the ones with higher disposable income and hence a good target market for these companies.

In the days since liberalization Gyms, Clinics, Supplements and diets have grown manifold. A recent quest for a personal instructor by my wife saw numerous coaches show up at our doorstep, some with their own assistants.

But what about the hungry kids? This situation of malnutrition is leading to be a stumbling block to India's progress in the long run with disease, disability and economic backwardness on the horizon for almost 20 % of India's future.

India continues to grapple with the problem of inadequate nutrition. The problem is more acute with children across stratum of society in this nation. On one hand we have children in some economic strata, who don't have access to a balanced diet due to the economic condition of the parents. They depend on the mid-day meal provided by the school or cheaper carbohydrates laden diet that is cheaper and something their parents can afford.

On the other end of the spectrum are children like my daughter who are over exposed to marketing from various FMCG companies and love to snack on carbohydrates laden diet. In our case we have introduced the concept of a balanced diet early on and thankfully my daughter seems to balancing her fondness for snacks with fruits.

Knowing all this it is important for parents to think through the nutritional intake of their children and focus on the lost growth. Before we jump into that you might be wondering how do you measure the growth of your child against the health standards prescribed by the Indian Medical Association (IMA) and the World Health Organization (WHO)

These are some other aspects

I think it is very important for children across India to balance their diet and catch up on the lost growth. These are some key facts

- Most children grow till the age of 18-21. In most cases this is the last growth spurt for height before the epiphyseal plates close on the long bones and there can be no more increase in height normally.

- In India by World Bank estimates 60 million children are malnourished, this means they don't have the right balance between carbohydrates, minerals, vitamins, proteins, water and fats. This nutritional deficiency affects them in various ways and eventually leads to issues like mineral deficiency, hormonal dysfunction, obesity, muscle pains, skeletal disorders and mental ill health. The number of 60 million also hides the number of malnourished children in the affluent families who risk losing growth due to lack of proteins. Add to this the new issues like Vitamin D Deficiency and Thyroid that accumulate due to our lifestyle of staying indoors.

- It is estimated that India has around 50 Million diabetics and this is spreading at such an alarming rate that it is tied back in most cases to nutritional imbalance as children. Most diabetic patients are unable to adjust to new lifestyle. Some researches in the west have found that bypass patients go back to old lifestyle 9 out of 10 times knowing that it is the lifestyle that got them into trouble in the first place. Also the adding sugar to the diet has created further complication as most diets and processed foods have added sugar.

- The age group of 3-9 years is the most crucial age group in India. Most Indian diets are rich in carbohydrates and lack in proteins. The situation is slightly worse in the otherwise healthy vegetarian diet. As children are attracted to tasty or instant food, it is impossible to feed them protein only through egg white or soy milk. Milk enabled nutritional supplements is definitely a solution in this space

So what can we do?

- Educate yourself, understand what you are eating and how it affects the health for you and family. Also this education will help you make informed buying decisions when in the market.

- Encourage the mid-day meal schemes started by some of the government schools. The novel idea was the brainchild of the former Tamilnadu chief minister M G Ramachandran. This resulted in increased literacy and also improved nourishment. Today as most schools are shut, the onus is back on the parents to provide for diet for children. But this remains the corner stone for our fight against malnutrition.

- Contribute to institutions like Akshay Patra. The Akshay Patra foundation has been the leading voice on nutrition. They run schemes to feed under privileged children. I am not saying we need to contribute to them only there are other NGOs working in the field, but Akshay Patra is the largest provider to the Mid-Day Meals for the children.

- Encourage the local community programs on nutrition. A good place is to start with the focus on domestic helps and their wards ensuring they have a balanced diet and educate them on it as well. Now this can be done from home itself, all you need to do is to start from your domestic helps and then spread it at the apartment and block level.

Unfortunately, there are no quick fixes for the malnutrition issue. It is a deep socio-economic problem but a beginning has to be made somewhere and it is better to start late rather than not start at all.

Well if we thought that children were our biggest concern, worry not. On the other end of the spectrum we have malnutrition affecting the elderly as well. As the years roll by, life seems to go full circle, and we find ourselves taking care of and worrying about those parents and elderly relatives who took care of and worried about us in our childhood. Ironically, one of the biggest individual concerns also goes full circle – trying to encourage them to eat the right things and get all the nutrients they need. Recent research published by Department of Community Medicine, Gauhati Medical College provided the shocking statistic that 15 percent of 360 senior citizens assessed in the study were suffering from malnutrition.

A healthy and nutritious diet is critical for seniors who want to remain mentally and physically healthy. The trouble is, many senior citizens suffer from a poor appetite, and in a country where a large proportion of the community is vegetarian, and there are extra considerations when it comes to providing adequate nutrition for our elderly. However, it is not as difficult as you might think. Here we take a look at three of the most important nutrients for the elderly.

Potassium

Potassium has a whole host of benefits. It is great for strong bones, which is essential for the elderly in the prevention of conditions such as osteoporosis, and also helps to regulate blood pressure. Potassium can also be found in a variety of everyday vegetables and fruits, including potatoes (especially the skins), bananas, prunes and plums.

Folic acid

Most people associate folic acid with expectant mothers, but it is also hugely important for the elderly, having been shown to significantly reduce the symptoms of dementia. It occurs naturally in green leafy vegetables including broccoli, spinach and peas.

Calcium

Another famous mineral, but perhaps one more associated with children, as it is great for teeth and bones. As we mentioned earlier, though, this is also an important consideration in the elderly, who are more prone to osteoporosis. Everyone knows that milk is a great source of calcium, but it can also be found in many green vegetables, including spinach, kale and broccoli.

Taking care of loved ones

The circularity of life can sometimes seem a little sad, but we should cherish the opportunity to repay the love and care we received in our formative years. Follow the above tips to provide the nutrition your elderly loved ones' need, and enjoy these special years together.

But in addition to this going by where we land with sedentary lifestyles and staying indoors most of the time it is important to keep a check on Vitamin D and Thyroid levels as discussed in the previous sections. Now let's look at another component of our lives, work-life balance.

Work Life Balance to Rejuvenate the Happiness Hormones

The other aspect of lifestyle that we often try to understand is flexible work timings. While many experts have written about flexible work timings and how it really impacts a person's mental and physical wellbeing, I think what is under our control is to set a very specific timetable framework in order to do work, when we are less distracted.

So, I am not going to tell you how you can increase your productivity because I think that is a very individualistic concept. Because what works for one person may not work for another person. But at the same time, I would highly recommend you set aside certain part of the day, which is distraction free, where you do your most critical work, and then batch your phone calls and meetings together. That way you can make the most out of your time in the day.

In one of my discussions with Dr. Sudhakar Varanasi he brought up an interesting statement, "When we replace the word 'I' with the word 'We', the word 'Illness' transforms to the word 'Wellness'." He attributes this quote to this father. This brings into focus the importance of social interactions. This is in line with the longest longitudinal study conducted by Harvard on 268 sophomore students started in 1938, and continued for 80 years, which gives us insights into health and happiness. Social interactions, meeting people, relationships are the keys to health. It works better than achievement and delays the mental and physical decline.

The other lifestyle change I would want you to consider is to reduce your digital media interactions. I think the Covid 19 pandemic has again forced us to avoid face to face contact and our social interactions have gone down tremendously. But at the same time compensating it by spending a lot of time on social media and digital media is a very bad idea from a health perspective.

So, your flexibility in your work style should also include digital free time in the day where you don't look at digital media. And instead focus on maybe reading a book or even a phone call to an old friend whom you haven't spoken in a while.

In the mental health section, we do talk about reconnecting with older friends as a great way to rejuvenate your mind and to keep your mental balance. I think Similarly, a great deal of your work life flexibility will come from your ability to reconnect with those from your past whom you haven't been in touch with. And due to your lifestyle and commute and work timings have not been able to connect.

So ideally, this is how I will divide my day. Spend some time for your physical activity, spend some time on your work, set aside some digital free time where you do creative work or you read a book or educate yourself and give some time to reconnect with those who you haven't spoken to of late because that really generates a spark and leaves you better than you are. I know there are you know hormonal impact and there is a lot of your you know dopamine as well as some of the hormones that are triggered because of you know these physical factors and they go a long way in keeping your mental balance.

Below is a table of the key hormones that affect your happiness and how you can boost them

Hormone	Natural Boosting Mechanism
Dopamine	Protein rich diet, exercise, music, adequate sleep
Seratonin	Sunlight, Massage, Exercise, Happy Events
Norepinephrine	Exercise, Cold Showers, Adequate Sleep
Endorphins	Exercise, Meditation, Aroma Therapy, Laughter
Melatonin	Sunlight, Adequate Sleep, Reduced Stress and limited Caffeine intake

Diagram 17 The key hormones and their effect on happiness, as you can see exercise and sleep are the key

As you can see from the list, a balanced diet, exercise, adequate sleep, and exposure to sunlight are the common factors for naturally triggering these hormones. That's why these are the key areas that we have tackled in this book in order to give you a natural boost to take care of your health. Let's look at sleep in more detail.

Sleep Management

It is believed that more than 90% of urban Indians don't get proper sleep, the numbers vary depending on the survey you refer to. But the key is that and we are sleeping less than what we earlier.

Very interestingly, Doug Reed, the founder of Netflix said their biggest competition was sleep. So, they're competing against your sleep, and he couldn't have said it better.

Whatever the reason might be, the fact that you are sleeping less is pretty evident- we are busy on OTT platforms, we are busy watching the internet, binge watching streaming video and web series that have no end. There is no logical stop to these episodes and often one episode starts even before the credits of the previous one ends, that's why most of these activities are so dangerous and addictive.

If we sleep later that means, we wake up later in the day. and the cycle goes on. And as work from home has permeated all parts of our life. In COVID-19, extended work from home has spurred the sleep disorders, getting worse as we borrow, our day perpetually from the next day. And we are in a continuous loop, in which we are unable to put an end to it.

Well, before you get panicky about the whole situation, I think the easiest thing to do is to shut down digital media before you go to sleep. Maybe an ideal time to do that will be around nine o'clock in the evening so that by 9 to 10 pm, you're in the dark, you're not watching any screens, allowing your body and mind to fall into sleep naturally.

I believe we need about 8 hours of sleep per day alongside a one-hour pre sleep ritual where we can wind down for the day. I think that should be enough. As we have seen earlier. Sleep is essential to a lot of the hormones that instil a sense of happiness to drive our sense of happiness and sleep is very important.

Owing to our busy lifestyles and hectic schedule, we avoid taking care of ourselves and health takes a backseat. Snoring, lack of sleep, if untreated can lead to an increased risk of severe medical conditions depression which can further lead to life threating health issues like diabetes, weight gain, high blood pressure and irregular heartbeat.

We have already seen that one of the biggest keys to happiness is adequate sleep. In India, 93% of the populations is sleep-deprived, but only 2% Indian discuss their sleep issues with physicians. The prevalence of Obstructive Sleep Apnoea (OSA) is high in Western India. So if you are in Mumbai, Pune or Ahmedabad please pay attention.

If you have issues going to sleep at night or have excessive sleepiness in the day, do discuss the same with your physician. Ancient Indian practices have laid a lot of importance on sleep. According to Ayurveda, the best time to go to bed is right around, or just before, 10:00 p.m., when Kapha gives way to Pitta. And it is important to get about 7-8 hours of sleep daily.

There are some conditions like insomnia, which are driven by sentiments. Jetlag is one of the biggest causes of insomnia. But today as we are traveling less that one element is ruled out. There are other conditions like obstructive sleep apnoea and central sleep apnoea. A lot of it is related to stress and obesity. But I would recommend before you take any decisions on these areas, please consult a physician. I always insist on it as there are many dangers of self-medication. Let us discuss that in some more detail.

The Dangers of Self Medication

A few days ago I was speaking to a friend over phone. Her voice was quivering and I could make out that she was unwell. On further inquiry I gathered that she had chills, fever, pain in the back and joints. On hearing this I was naturally worried as these are some of the symptoms of Dengue. I recommended that she meet a doctor immediately. She was reluctant to go as she had already taken some fever medication. But I still insisted and she finally did visit a doctor. Luckily for her, she tested negative for Malaria and Dengue, but she still had infection and the doctor prescribed the necessary antibiotics.

The incident got me to think about the state of self-medication in the country. In 2015 an online portal had asked more than 20,000 respondents questions around medication. More than 50% respondents had resorted to self-medication that year. I am not surprised at the number. The most common reasons given by the respondents were the exorbitant fees at private clinics, long lines at government run hospitals and the reluctance of the patients to get diagnostic tests done.

I usually take online surveys with a pinch of salt as most people do tend to lie on such surveys. According to a study conducted among 352 patients in Puducherry across 124 households it was found that prevalence of self-medication was found to be 11.9%. Males over 40 years involved in moderate level activity were found to be significantly associated with higher self-medication usage. Fever (31%), headache (19%), and abdominal pain (16.7%) are most common illnesses where self-medication is being used. Telling the symptoms to the pharmacist (38.1%) was the commonest method adopted to procure drugs by the users. Majority of the self-medication users expressed that self-medication is harmless (66.6%) and they are going to use (90%) and advice others also (73.8%) to use self-medication drugs.

I think the numbers are more realistic here, but again regional variation could change all that. I would expect the numbers to be higher in the north and the east of the country and lower in south and west.

Another exploratory study conducted by Greenhalgh T studied the drugs supplied to 2400 patients by the public and private medical sectors and by private pharmacies. These were supplied based on patient complaints on illness and subsequent prescriptions from the doctors. The most interesting finding of the study was the private sector was prescribing more drugs than the government run hospitals. Many of these drugs were combination preparation (Medical Cocktails) and also contained some hidden classes of drugs.

Prescription medicine was being sold over the counter; some very powerful medicines were being prescribed for simple conditions. Also many drugs banned in the west were still being prescribed in India. Another interesting finding was that food supplements and tonics of dubious nutritional and pharmacological value made up a high proportion of the total drugs bill.

The study also concluded that any drug policy from the government might have to involve doctor and pharmacist education to reduce the over prescription of drugs.

There are many dangers of self-medication. Apart from side effects and ill effects, most public health experts feel that it leads to long term challenges like

1. Drug resistance, this is the biggest challenge in our fight against TB for example. Ciprofloxacin prescribed for throat infections is also an anti-TB drug

2. Allergies, as most of these combination medicines with hidden classes of drugs are notorious for causing allergies

3. Late diagnosis – If self- medication is the first line of attack, often by the time the patient reaches the doctor it is often late. Late diagnosis leads to late treatment, delayed recovery and more medical bills.

In my opinion please consider the following:

1. Stop self-medication immediately.

2. Visit your doctor in case of any symptoms. If you don't have a family doctor then, identify a good family medicine practitioner in your neighbourhood and visit him regularly.

3. Today with Telemedicine it is very simple and convenient to set up an online consultation, and medicines are being delivered home through online pharmacies.

4. Maintain all your medical records; there are apps that can help you with it, otherwise just keep a file if you are not tech savvy. Scanning and uploading records to Google Drive is also a good option. But there are privacy concerns around it so be very careful with your records.

If you have the time to visit the mall or the hairdresser regularly, then visiting the doctor should not be such a painful experience. In the end if you see it is our mind-set that needs to change. Mind-set needs to change everywhere, and the Indian Healthcare system is no different.

Genetics – From one generation to another

While we have discussed a lot about health and the various parameters of health, the one area of health that is very less understood is genetics. Genetics is the genetic code that runs you. You are you because of your genetic code.

As I said you are because of your genetic code, and Genetic research studies have now shown that individual genes or various genes that are involved within you are involved in a lot of health and disease factors. Understanding genetic code and disease factors is very important and today with the advancement of technology, we have been able to break down what your genetic code actually stands for, and also can identify what risks one is prone to.

Unfortunately, genetics is not entirely under your control. I have always said your health is in your hands, all the factors that have said before, this can be controlled in some form or fashion. Except your genes. But you can do with your genes of course is to understand what are you predisposed to and put in some controls or some monitoring factors that will help you manage health issues.

A good example was what an actress did some years ago, when she understood that she carried a gene that was present in her mother, which would eventually increase the risk of breast cancer for her. She attacked it progressively and underwent a mastectomy, just to make sure that that issue did not arise with her. Anybody who's been in a science class in school would know that we have 46 chromosomes, 23 pairs. We receive half our chromosomes from our father and the other half from Mother.

If you're a man you received a Y chromosome from your father and a X chrome from your mother. If you are a woman then you received an X chromosome from your mother and an X chromosome from your father. Now a lot of the genetic disorders, often come when the chromosome gets passed on from one parent to the child. That means you are more predisposed to anything that your parents have been carrying. Now there are two gene forms here.

One is called a dominant gene and the other is called a recessive gene, a dominant gene is something that is dominating you, that means if your father had a condition and that chromosome is dominating in you then you will definitely have it. It could be a recessive gene in which you become a carrier. And so, If your parents had a disease, and that gene is dominant in you, there's a 50% chance of you inheriting the gene. But if it's a recessive gene there is a 25% chance of a disease or carrying the gene. That means, you might become a carrier, but not show any symptoms. There are also many single gene disorders.

There are a lot of labs in India that do your genetic mapping, it is not very expensive these days to go through it. It will be great, just to give a sample of your saliva, or some DNA, for them to analyse your genetic code and see what conditions you are predisposed to. There are a few examples that I've seen globally.

One is, obviously, this can be used to identify breast cancer, Also in certain conditions. You can also identify heart conditions. You cannot change, but you can definitely identify what are the risk factors for you and take some precautions.

Coronary Heart Disease is a lethal condition which affects 30 million people in India. Last year there were almost 2,00,000 heart surgeries performed in the country. Traditionally doctors treating Coronary Heart Disease look for certain facts including

1.   Cholesterol Level

2.   High Blood Pressure

3.   Smoking

4.   Diabetes

These 4 factors were the key to identify patients at risk. But these are very broad based and not very effective in identifying patients most at risk for coronary heart disease. As you may know, the symptoms of coronary heart disease, which may include, Chest pain or Angina, Pain in the muscles, joints and shoulders, shortness of breath, indigestion. Most of these symptoms are exaggerated by work or effort and come down with rest. They also sometimes are triggered by emotional outbursts. In most cases early detection and intervention is the key to a successful treatment for coronary heart disease.

Physicians in Leicester University in the UK have come up with a Genome Risk Score. Our genes predetermine conditions like Coronary Heart Disease and mostly small variations on the DNA can dramatically change outcomes. So a Single Nucleotide Polymorphism or SNP can determine the exact risk of developing coronary heart disease. Scientists studies more than 40,000 SNPs to come up with a Genomic Risk Score for Coronary Heart Disease. This when combined with the clinical risk factors stated earlier can help physicians ascertain those in most risk of developing coronary health disease. The higher the Genomic Risk Score the higher the future risk of Coronary Heart Disease. People with a Genomic Risk Score in the top 20 per cent had an over five-fold higher life-time risk of Coronary Heart Disease.

According to Professor Nilesh Samani at the University of Leicester in UK, this study shows the potential benefits of using a genetic risk score over and above current methods to identify people at increased risk of coronary heart disease. We already know that Coronary Heart Disease starts at an early age, several decades before symptoms develop, and preventative measures should ideally be applied much earlier, especially to those who are at increased risk. Dengue caused by Aedes Aegypti species is a dangerous condition and rampart urbanization and lack of planning has led to the disease spreading like wildfire in urban India.

In the past, in Healthcare India, we have covered various steps that can be tackled to manage the spread and growth of Dengue. We talked about insurance schemes that can help reduce the financial burden for families affected by Dengue and about how disease surveillance programs can help to reduce the spread of Dengue.

Genetic studies are also being used in the containment of Dengue.

In Maharashtra, the Gangabishan Bhikulal Trading Company (GBIT) has been working on leveraging genetics to handle the mosquito population responsible for the spread of Dengue. In 2008 they entered into an agreement with the UK based Bio Technology company Oxitec, which specializes in genetically modified insects. As part of the agreement GBIT has imported eggs of genetically modified Aedes Aegypti mosquitoes. Once these mosquitoes with the strain (OX513A) mate with the local females, the offspring then produced would never reach adulthood. This in their opinion would drastically reduce the population of the mosquito. And this would result in lowering the spread of Dengue across India.

In Puducherry (Formerly Pondicherry) the Vector Control Research Center the approach to Dengue is slightly different. Indian Council of Medical Research (ICMR) is working in collaboration with Monash University to introduce bacteria infected mosquito cells from Australia.

The bacteria in the cells would work in two ways

- It would improve the immunity of the Aedes Aegypti mosquito so that the Dengue virus finds it difficult to infect the mosquito

- Also, the Bacteria will compete with the virus for the resources in the mosquito's body and limit the spread of the virus.

In both instances the incidents of Dengue should come down.

Interesting concepts and hopefully one of these approaches will get us results. In the past, there have been pilots in eradicating the malaria mosquito in a similar fashion in the 1970's. But due to mixed results the pilots never continued.

In addition to genetics there is an effort to develop a vaccine for Dengue. Dengvaxia by Sanofi Pasteur has been approved in more than 20 countries and is waiting for approval in India. There is also an indigenous vaccine being developed by the International Center for genetic engineering and bio technology.

In 2018 UK-based genomics data platform Global Gene Corp and American genetics company, Regeneron Genetics Center announced that they will collaborate to create the world's largest project of its kind to study Indian population.

The multi-year-tie-up is aimed at finding innovative diagnosis and therapies for rare diseases. Genomic sequencing data generated by Regeneron Research Center will be paired with de-identified medical records from consenting patients to examine links between human genetic variations and disease. Global Gene Corp is founded by my classmate Sumit Jamuar and hopefully this project will reveal more about our genes and how to prevent diseases.

Own Your Health – what you can do

Well in summary below is the framework that is populated for your benefit.

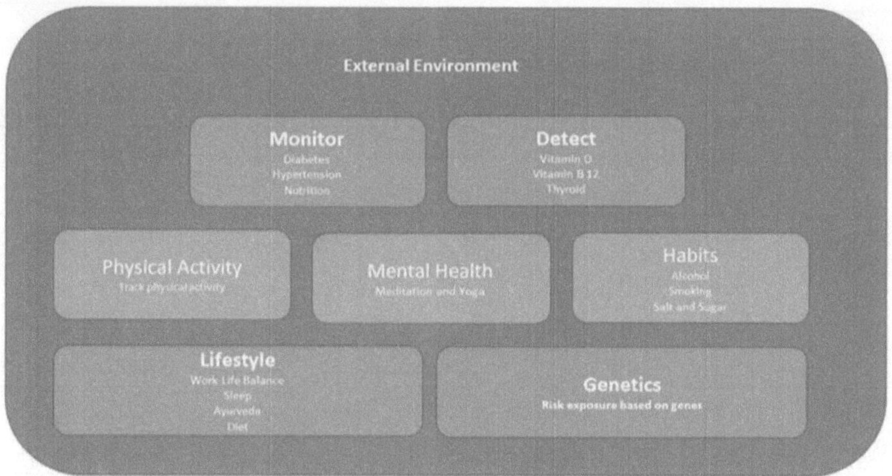

Diagram 18 The Own your Health Framework Populated with the key parameters

I have also added this as a chart as part of the framework that you can track.

	What	**How**	**Frequency**	**Method**
Monitor	Diabetes	Random Blood Sugar	Monthly	Home Glucometer
	Diabetes	HbA1c	Quarterly	Lab
	Hypertension	Blood Pressure	Weekly	Home Blood Pressure Monitor, Smart Watch
	Nutrition	Food Intake	Daily	Mobile App
Detect	Vitamin D	Serum Vitamin D levels	Quarterly	Lab
	Vitamin B 12	Serum Vitamin B 12 Levels	Quarterly	Lab
	Thyroid	TSH, T3 and T4 levels	Quarterly	Lab
Physical Activity	Track exercise- Walk, Sports Etc	Monitor Movement	Daily	Mobile App, Fitness Tracker, Smart Watch
Mental Wellness	Meditation,	Meditation Time	Daily	Mobile App, Smart Watch
	Yoga	Practice Time	Daily/ Weekly	Mobile App, Smart Watch
Habits	Alcohol	Number of Drinks	Daily/As Applicable	Mobile App
	Smoking	Number of Cigarettes	Daily /As Applicable	Mobile App
	Salt	Salt Intake	Daily	Mobile App
	Sugar	Sugar Intake	Daily	Mobile App
Lifestyle	Diet	Calorie Intake	Daily	Mobile App
	Sleep	Sleep Pattern and Duration	Daily	Mobile App

	Work life Balance	Work life Balance	Daily	Mobile App
	Ayurveda	Daily / Weekly Concoction if applicable	As applicable	Mobile App
Genetics	Risk predisposition to other diseases	Check for Risk Factors	Lifetime once	Lab

SECTION 2
The Healthcare Industry

How patient experience is driving healthcare

As you know in January 30, 2020, India recorded its first case for Corona Virus popularly known as Covid19. Since then India has seen a series of lockdowns and as we inch towards somewhat of a partial recovery, the question around the state of our healthcare system has become centre stage again.

Since the 1940's where the Bhore committee gave its recommendations for developing the healthcare structure in India, as a nation we have been playing catch up with demand far exceeding the supply in terms of doctors, diagnostic equipment, hospital beds and medicines.

In addition, wellness programs have been struggling and preventive measures have not been very successful. In this context the corner stone of the healthcare system in India has become the hospital.

What determines a successful healthcare intervention is patient experience. Today with the advent of telehealth and the guidelines given by Medical Council of India, it becomes even more important for hospitals to focus on patient experience and add to the growth of the industry.

Private hospitals have long tracked patient satisfaction ratings, but they didn't always carry great significance. While all hospitals want happy patients, most hospitals have been historically plagued with the "doctor knows best" mentality — a mentality where clinical outcomes outweigh "touchy-feely" indicators such as patient satisfaction or overall patient experience.

However, in recent years, some leading institutions in India have begun to focus more heavily on providing an outstanding patient experience. Drivers for this include growing consumerism and transparency for healthcare services and increased interest from both consumers and providers in patient-centred care.

Healthcare consumers increasingly view their experience with a provider as a key consideration for determining if they'll return to or recommend the provider, largely because it remains one of the few ways consumers can differentiate providers. Over the past few decades, clinical outcomes have improved dramatically, and patients no longer view favourable outcomes as a key differentiator as these are expected. What remains is the patient's overall experience, which encompasses everything from customer service to patient-centeredness and care coordination among providers. Also given the growth of Tele Health, it would become even more important for hospitals to focus on patient experience in order to create a favourable experience and create the hook that would bring patients and others in the community back to the hospital.

While there are many parameters that determine patient experience, we have tried to list down a few key ones that might influence the satisfaction index more than the others.

1. Patient Appointment Experience

2. Patient Online Portal

3. Social Media and Digital Out Reach

4. Facility for the In-Patient Service and Emergency Service

5. Patient's Access to medical Records

6. Patient Information

7.   Clinical Outcomes

8.   Value Added Service

Following are the key digital parameters for patient experience at major Indian Hospitals:

1.   Video consultation with consultants- Telemedicine

2.   Online Appointment System

3.   Mobile Application

4.   Internal Navigation

5.   Online digital Payment method

6.   Health Library with A-Z medical information

7.   Digital Helpline- Online 24*7 Expert Opinion

8.   Virtual tour of the Hospital

Accessibility and affordability along with quality healthcare are the main issues when it comes to medical treatment in Indian hospitals. When a patient visits a hospital he/she expects all the services wanted at ease but unfortunately they can face a lot of issues of medical negligence, casual approach at various department starting from the registration to OPD, check up to billing. To curb these problem hospitals are currently emphasizing on digitalization for the better patient experience. One of the major revolutionary step towards it is providing telehealth or telemedicine services. This can not only save the cost of the treatment but can give the patients a comfortable homely atmosphere at a healthcare setting. But there should be a balance between both physical and digital experience at the hospital. In a country like India, many people are still sceptical about adopting technology properly, for them it still what they experience after reaching the hospital. So hospitals should implement digital services like implementing telemedicine, Electronic Health Record, Mobile Health etc. but they should also keep in mind the poor digital and IT literacy, low internet penetration, lack of regionally relevant content etc. So, improving of physical experience should also not be denied but both should be in well accord with each other for providing better healthcare to the patients.

Patient journey mapping is an exercise that healthcare marketers at hospitals can use to better understand what individuals experience throughout the entire patient journey. The patient journey map, which outlines all of the patient touch points during each stage of the care journey, aids in creating strategic outreach that improves both patient engagement and satisfaction.

The patient journey typically consists of six stages:

- Awareness of the condition: The patient self-assesses their conditions and symptoms, conducts research, and reaches out to online communities (posing questions on social media, etc.)

- Identify the right provider or specialist: The patient makes initial contact with a health system. This can be done via call centre, email, mobile, etc.

- Diagnosis: The patient is assessed at medical facility (physician's office, hospital,

- Treatment: The health system gives the patient on-site and follow-up care (medications, physical therapy, etc.)

- Behavioural/Lifestyle Change: The patient makes changes to their routines to reduce readmissions and promote proactive health

- Ongoing Care/Post-Operative Care: The patient manages their care between clinical visits. The health system fosters engagement between the patient & physicians to enable the patient to better manage his/her own care.

Using patient journey maps as guides, marketing managers of hospitals can craft strategic, personalized outreach that keeps patients engaged throughout the care journey, as well as implement programs that fill potential gaps in the care experience. Ultimately, patient journey maps help healthcare marketers improve patient engagement and foster lasting patient-provider relationships.

How Indian healthcare system is tackling diabetes

As discussed in the earlier part of the book, Diabetes is a resident pandemic in India, the only challenge is that it is a lifestyle condition and not a disease.

Diabetes is a major concern for India. Not only does it affect the individuals directly, but also accelerates the degeneration of nerves, blood vessels and tissues.

As we know India has around 50 million diabetics. But what would be interesting is that the condition is not new to India. Charaka, India's super physician has written about diabetes in his hallmark work Charaka Samhita. The management of diabetes is the key as there is no cure. One must constantly monitor blood sugar levels, diet and exercise. In other words, it is a constant process and needs expertise, advice, motivation and counselling. India has many diabetes managements centres. But Dr. Mohan's Diabetes Specialties Center was one of the first and still is a pioneer in Diabetes research. Founded in 1991, the research-based centre is the brain child of Dr. V Mohan, endocrinologist and pioneer in the field of diabetes research.

Diabetes management has been the corner stone of Dr. Mohan's family. His father, the Late Prof Dr. M Viswanathan, is widely recognized as India's first endocrinologist who specialized in Diabetes management. He joined Stanley Medical College in Madras (Now Chennai) in 1948 and was responsible for most of the research and the treatment modalities within the government sector at that time. For a long time, the medical institutions did not focus on diabetes management and it was only in 1973 that PGI Chandigarh started post-graduation in endocrinology with 2 seats in that space. The late Prof M Viswanathan continued his work at Stanley medical College till 1971 and then set up his own practice and opened MV Hospital and Diabetes Research Center in the northern part of Madras (Now Chennai).

It was here that Dr. Mohan joined his father. Dr. Mohan was in first year of MBBS and he used to help his father with research, setting up the laboratory and then helping him with his research papers. This way Dr. Mohan's focus was diabetes from the very beginning of his medical education as this is something rare in the field of medicine as most students decide on their super specialties at a much later stage.

This situation was unique, and Dr. Mohan travelled extensively with his father listening to his talks and interacting with other experts in the field of diabetes. In 1991 post his super specialization Dr. Mohan branched out on his own, setting up Dr. Mohan's Diabetes Specialties Center in south Madras (now Chennai). Here is where Dr. Mohan introduced what were considered new concepts in India like Computers, Modern Laboratory, Electronic medical records (EMR) and since then, they have been one of the first to adopt new technologies.

They started branches in Tamil Nadu, Hyderabad, Lucknow, Bhubaneshwar, Delhi and then now in Karnataka. They opened centers in Whitefiled, Malleswaram, Jaynagar, Mysore and Managlore.

In 2017 Dr. Mohan's Diabetes Specialty Center received private equity and that has helped the group standardize their offering and focus on diabetes care in an effective manner. Today the chain has 32 branches. So over the last 40 years and across 3 generations this chain has tracked, identified and managed Diabetes.

So I asked Dr. Mohan, what's so unique about his group. I know Diabetes is a challenge for India but how is their philosophy in management of Diabetes different from the others

Based on his responses, here is what I feel are the key investments that set Dr. V Mohan's center apart

- Research- They have been the pioneers and leaders in Diabetes research. The Madras Diabetes Research Foundation was set up by Dr. V Mohan in 1996. This is a 40,000 sq feet facility in Siruseri in Chennai. It is privately funded, staffed by 25 PHDs and 20 Post-Doctoral fellows with the sole intention of research in diabetes care and management. Through the foundation they have released more than 1000 research articles, peer reviewed in International and national journals in the field of diabetes. This foundation serves as a strong backbone of the Diabetes Specialties Center.

- As part of the research Dr. Mohan and his team have come up with practical solutions in areas like nutrition. So, the research is holistic. One of the solutions so developed is the High Fiber Rice, which has lower glycemic index and can be consumed by patients with diabetes. They have also brought other variants like high fiber "Rava". All these were possible due to the partnership with Department of Biotechnology in government of India.

- The Madras Diabetes Research Foundation has been training post-doctoral fellows for more than 20 years. This has helped them create a pool of diabetes specialists that have formed the core for the expansion of the group. As these doctors are well trained in the approach of running Diabetes management programs, the quality is maintained. A very good lesson for other organizations as they create future leaders that can help organizations grow in the future.

- They have also been leaders in technology, with being the first to introduce EMRs. The labs and the clinics are certified by ISO 9000, NABL and NABH respectively. In addition, they have collaboration with World Health Organization (WHO), Indian Council of Medical Research (ICMR) and National Institute of health (NIH)

Today Dr. Mohan's Diabetes Research Center has medical records of more than 5,00,000 patients across 25 years and it is probably the largest and longitudinally the longest database for diabetes research. Today they have probably all genotypes and phenotypes for India. And this helps them develop treatment modalities leveraging analytics which mines insights from their data.

I believe that super specialized centers like the one built by Dr. Mohan may be the key to managing some of the chronic non-communicable diseases in India. With the emphasis on research and adoption of technology, the future of Diabetes management in the country looks bright. But this is only the beginning.

Telemedicine – Anytime, Anywhere Consultation

Telemedicine is the delivery of healthcare consultancy, advice and treatment guidelines over technology, negating the need for the patient and doctor to be co-located. It is the extension of how we work in virtual teams, connected by internet and telephony.

What makes Tele-Medicine a necessity in India is the distribution of the Indian population, 70 % of which is spread over 700,000 villages in India, most with population less than 1000 people. The second factor necessitating the need for Tele-Medicine in India is the lack of doctors and trained nurses. If current estimates are believed there is a short fall of 600,000 doctors in India. To add to it now we have low cost portable monitoring device like the $ 100 Ultra Sound developed by GE. Finally we have the wide spread reach of mobile communication, where India has more mobile phones than toilets.

When I was a practicing dentist, I would often receive telephone calls from my friends and relatives for advice on their dental problems. I have also analysed and studied X rays sent over MMS and SMS and given diagnosis. So I was way into Tele-medicine space before it was established as a practice. Even today my colleagues give advice and prescriptions to their patients over phone for non-critical symptoms.

But the challenge remains can doctors make money by consulting over phone? Because the basis of capitalism is getting compensated for effort otherwise the idea does not take off.

One of the perplexing questions that have baffled technologists for long is why regulators have not approved the use of teleconsultation for doctors. In the past, I have felt the need for Tele-Consultation or Telemedicine, to improve care in India.

Here are my reasons

1. As a doctor, I used to see the 8 hours of practice work as heavily imbalanced. I was free for the first 5 hours of the day but loaded towards the evening. The last three hours and especially the weekends would be packed and I would be overworking at that time. If I had to balance that time well, I would have liked to equally distribute the patients throughout the 8 hours. But as I would have to meet the patients and they might require someone to bring them to the clinics.

2. Our health infrastructure, both in terms of people, beds and devices, is based in the cities. Our rural areas are underserved and they need to make the trip to the cities for any healthcare service. Sometimes even to take a blood test or an X-Ray. While they might need to make the trip to avail of lab facilities, through Tele Medicine, the consultation problem should be solved.

3. India needs cheap access to care. Most consultations are expensive as they take into account the investments in infrastructure, rent, etc. With Telemedicine, one has to only pay rent for platform and bandwidth charges. The overall cost of consultation should come down.

While many in the industry including me have argued for this for long, the regulations until recently did not allow for telemedicine or teleconsultation.

The breakout of Covid19 changed everything. With social distancing emerging as the best defence against Covid19 it is obvious that the next step was the guidelines for telemedicine from the Medical Council of India.

On 25th March 2020, the Medical Council of India along with Niti Aayog released the Telemedicine Practice Guidelines.

In summary, these are the key areas covered by the document.

1. Guidelines for Telemedicine in India Elements specific to Telemedicine

    - Appropriateness of Telemedicine

    - Identification of RMP and the patient

    - Appropriateness of technology/Mode of Telemedicine

    - Patient Consent · Patient Evaluation · Patient Management: Health education, counselling and medication Duties and responsibilities of RMP in general

    - Medical Ethics, Data Privacy & Confidentiality

    - Documentation and Digital Records of Consultation

    - Fee for Telemedicine

2. Framework for Telemedicine

    - Patient to Registered Medical Practitioner

    - Care Giver to Registered Medical Practitioner

    - Patient to RMP through Health Worker at a Sub Center or any peripheral center

    - Registered Medical Practitioner to another RMP / Specialist

3. Guidelines for Technology Platforms enabling Telemedicine

I would recommend that everyone should read these guidelines. It's a great read for start-ups and technology providers planning to build these platforms and healthcare providers planning to develop their telemedicine services. So now you have one less excuse to self-medicate, making it much easier to consult a qualified doctor. Now let's see what you can expect from your hospitals in terms of technology adoption and digital transformation.

Indian hospitals are adopting technology faster than before

Is Healthcare ready to adopt technology?

This is the largest question that we faced since liberalisation. Finally, in 2020 we have adopted technology like never before in healthcare. Telemedicine adoption is increasing, contact tracing through healthcare applications is the norm. But having said this let's look at the historical context in India and let me take you back to a discussion I hosted some years ago on this topic.

In the ancient times India had family healers that were called upon to combat disease and improve the standards of care. These medicine men of the old not only had knowledge of fields like Ayurveda, Siddha and Unani but also had knowledge of family history that used to help in their diagnosis. After the coming of the British though traditional medicine got supplanted by modern allopathic treatment, the role of the family physician continued. So family history and your medical history was known to these physicians. In a sense we had an efficient system for Big Data and Analytics though it was not system driven. But healthcare till then was the privilege of a few and not easily available to all.

With the breakdown of the joint family system and the mass migration to the cities since independence, we see that the family physicians are hard to come by. While healthcare is more available in the cities, most patients prefer specialists and as a result, the medical history is lost. For example, you have an eye irritation so you would go to an ophthalmologist, who would prescribe a few medicines and solve the problem. Subsequently a couple of years later if you have the same eye irritation you might not have saved the previous prescription or scanned it on, to create a digitized copy, as a result the new doctor would not know your history.

As a result of this issue, the west has embraced Big Data and Analytics in a big way. In the US for example, most hospital systems would have your medical history and even if you switch physicians, your health insurance firm would have your history. In the UK the NHS has health records on all your ailments and also has records on your family history if they lived in the UK. In both these scenarios the adoption of technology has also led to increased investments in areas like Big Data and Analytics. Hospitals are able to predict patterns for re admission for other patients and are able to institute preventive measures to ensure against it. Also use of analytics helps them understand disease patterns in the community and focus on population health initiatives to improve the health standards of a community.

According to Rajesh Batra, CIO Kokilaben Hospital, the task at the moment is to face our fears about the future with courage. we need to turn to technologies with an open mind and prepare for the changing world with as much knowledge as possible. Digital technology (hopefully will be the panacea) could help transform unsustainable healthcare into a sustainable one, and be the equalizer for the relationship between medical professionals and patients and provide the bridge for cheaper, faster and more effective solution.

But in India with technology adoption in the hospitals just at the inception, what is the future for adoption of big data and analytics?

As part of various industry committees, I have led these discussions, drafted policies and submitted papers to the industry as well as to the government. While the National Digital Health Blue Print has been launched, it is still a long way off from setting the framework for analytics and big data in the industry.

There are a number of reasons for the same. Firstly, it is very difficult to get any kind of analysis going with the hospital systems today. Paper records take time to be digitized and by the time they can get any analysis going for patient readmission or population health monitoring it is almost 6 months. While most people felt doctors did not like digital or adopt them faster, the truth is far from it. But improved digital form factors could definitely enhance the adoption of big data among medical professionals.

Most doctors would like to look at the patient while they are writing prescriptions, an art most doctors have perfected over the years, but the same cannot be said about typing into the device. So, innovation must come in while deciding the form factor of the devices and systems used in the healthcare set up. Clearly it is up to the UX and design community to help doctors adopt analytics and big data and improve its adoption in Indian healthcare set up.

Areas like understanding the disease patterns and evaluating doctor load is another area where analytics has been used. Patient satisfaction surveys which were taken a few days into admission of the patient and if any concerns found were acted upon almost immediately. When the surveys were re-administered, both patients and their party polled higher on satisfaction. So analytics in a way helped the hospital to respond to feedback real time unlike the traditional model where it would have taken days or even weeks to act upon surveys.

I have been using HealthfyMe for a while and behind the app is an analytics engine that has been running. HealthifyMe worked with the department of nutrition, government of India to classify more than 10 million Indian food items, that was a mammoth task by itself and a huge

Big Data project, but since then they have users creating content and the speed and agility of user created content has been phenomenal.

Also the Indian big data and analytics issues can be divided into two parts, dealing with legacy data and the new age user created data. The two need different systems to deal with.

Philips has been doing a lot of work in this space, looking at technology from a patient perspective has given those options to partner with organizations to deliver improved care on the backbone of analytics and big data. Incidentally Manipal Health Ventures, Philips Healthcare and HealthifyMe have joined hands to work on a wellness program for the employees.

Located in a bustling road at the heart of Bangalore, Manipal Hospital is not new to technology.

In 2015, they became the first hospital in India, and among the first few in the world, to adopt IBM's Watson platform for oncology diagnosis.

In a recent study conducted by the hospital involving 600-plus breast cancer cases, it was observed that concordance between the recommendations provided by Watson and that by the Manipal Hospital's oncologists was as high as 90%.

This means patients now have the advantage of seeking diagnosis from the Watson platform, in addition to a specialist oncologist at the hospital.

The Watson platform was tutored on the cases by accessing clinical data of patients already treated at Manipal. All cases considered in the study were approved by the scientific committee and the ethics committee constituted by the hospital, before being fed into the Watson platform.

Manipal Hospital has also been analysing its Health Information System (HIS) data, particularly on the progression of kidney diseases in patients. On comparing Kidney Function Test parameters between patients in India and patients in the West, it was found that the rate of kidney deterioration in a Caucasian diabetic patient was 1% but that in an Indian diabetic patient was 4%. This helped the hospital devise a program for early intervention in diabetic patients in India.

As we can see from above healthcare ecosystem is poised for a massive digital transformation. In coming times, doctors will rely more on technology in addition to the knowledge augmented by human contact. Path-breaking technologies like AI and cognitive solutions will potentially transform the care continuum and alter patient's experience. Hospitals are increasingly embracing digital solutions and relying more on technology. Not only large hospitals but startups have joined the fray as well. Investments in health-tech start-ups have exhibited significant growth in the last 3 years. One such indigenous health-technology startup is Niramai, which uses machine intelligence to detect and diagnose breast cancer using thermographic images. It has developed a low cost, non-contact, non-invasive and radiation-free breast cancer screening solution which can detect tumors that are five times smaller than what can be detected through a clinical examination. This help in early detection of breast cancer and hence improves the survival rate. Another India based startup, Qure.ai, uses artificial intelligence to provide automated interpretation of MRI & CT scans and X-Rays. One of its tool – to analyse head CT scans- has received FDA proposal and can identify potential stoke or head injury. The model has been constantly improved by using 1 million X-rays and their reports.

In my opinion a lot more work needs to be done as these are just point solutions. Yes, we need these insights and they have to come from the medical history but the way we are structured I don't think it will be anytime soon that we would be able to leverage the full benefits of big data and analytics on the Indian healthcare scenario

These are some of my insights and guidance for greater adoption of technology

1. Form factor or User Interface and better User Experience is the key to the adoption of technology by the doctors

2. We definitely require analytics but on Big Data I reserve my opinion. It would require a lot of ground work and currently we are not in a position to launch Big Data in Healthcare

3. Hospitals have started adoption these technologies on the patient satisfaction front and organizations are coming together to engage on employee wellness initiatives

4. The future of adoption belongs to start ups and how they can think innovatively and introduce new ideas that would use these technologies to improve care models in India

So while most people in the community will benefit from this, it is up to the citizens to also think of ways of improving the form factors and adoption of technology for the same. Technology adoption is important and let's see why in the subsequent chapters. Especially in areas like disease surveillance.

Why Disease Surveillance will help improve citizen health services

India is perhaps the only country in the world (of its size) where addressing preventable diseases continues to drain public resources. The Delhi dengue outbreak in 2017 is a case in point. This is the third or fourth time in a decade (the first being in 2006) that the city has failed to prevent the spread of this disease. Close to 3,500 cases of dengue have been reported in Delhi over that period, of which nearly all cases required hospitalization.

If the government wants to prevent such large-scale outbreak of disease in the future, it needs to consider leveraging disease surveillance systems that rely on digital/social media to inform, educate and warn citizens.

How a digital disease surveillance system can help?

A digital disease surveillance system collects data from multiple sources (in real time or otherwise) and can help indicate the potential of disease outbreak in certain locations, thereby enabling the government to take steps to control the situation.

Mature economies have been doing this for some time now and rely significantly on digital and social media to prevent and manage outbreaks. For instance, the US was able to identify cases of Ebola around 9 days before the World Health Organization declared the Ebola epidemic using a software that mines social media. This software, part of an infectious disease surveillance system, was able to pick up instances of a "mystery haemorrhagic fever" from among the various entries listed on government websites, local news sites, and social networks, correlating it with Ebola.

In other cases, it looked at the social media feed from users who indicated their ailments – directly (by looking at feed that saw people discussing their illness or indicating that they were unwell on social media) or indirectly (by analysing the number of people searching websites like Google, looking to investigate their symptoms and seek cure). This could have easily been applied to India, where we often self-medicate and hesitate to seek out professional medical help, unless one's health significantly deteriorates. Especially in cases like dengue, symptoms aren't unique enough to arouse suspicions from patients or their families to immediately seek medical help.

Another example is that of a disease detection app called Flu Near You. This app helps predict outbreaks of the flu in real time. Users self-report symptoms in a weekly survey, which the app then analyses and maps to show where pockets of influenza-like illness are located. Although there is an element of potential inaccurate reporting by citizens and the real possibility of symptoms not correlating with any specific disease (such as cold or headache may not directly help identify a serious condition), it is still a model that India could use in some areas where care is difficult to administer. The Aarogya Setu application on mobile phones used in fighting Covid19 is a similar application based on the same principles.

Integrating weather into disease surveillance

Some developed nations are also working on a more comprehensive disease monitoring mechanism that involves use of weather data. After all weather influences our health and any seasonal variations tend to bring about the bulk of diseases in the world.

Germany has been sharing 'health-weather' forecasting for three decades now. Newspapers not only carry the weather data, but also include information such as likely diseases accompanying the weather (up to 40 different diseases are covered) as well as symptoms (such as irritation, insomnia). On TV, varying degrees of symptoms and diseases are also provided. The website Wunderground.com, provides flu activity, pollen allergy and UV burns related information or Dachau in Germany. Media company AccuWeather now provides such health forecast for other countries too, like one focused on allergies in New York city.

Japan undertook health-weather forecasting by including Ultra Violet (UV) forecasting, adjusted to skin type as part of its surveillance mechanism in 2008. The country has been divided into 39 regions based on significant differences in terms of lifestyles, clothing, and sensibilities of residents. Each region sees certain variable such as heat, air temperature and humidity dominating public health. For each region, these unique parameters are considered before the weather-health forecast is put out. These forecasts can be obtained by any citizen with a mobile phone. Those visiting the website where these forecasts are made, have the option of sharing feedback which is then used to validate the forecast.

Britain's NHS piloted a health forecasting unit in 2001 that integrated weather data with infectious disease surveillance data in real time from five locations to help generate workloads prediction for those areas. For instance, flash warnings were given to ambulance services and accidents and emergency services units if the weather snowed or ice fell in anticipation of increased trauma and falls. Today this system has evolved to such an extent that hospitals prepare themselves for treating patients of heart and lung conditions that can worsen during cold weather. A comprehensive alert system has been set up and cold weather alerts are provided between November and April. A similar heat wave related alert system is also in place.

Considering the dengue outbreak in India first started in 2006 and has been recurring over the last 3-4 years involving similar casualties, the government could have used historical data to identify vulnerable areas and taken extra efforts to mitigate the risks this time.

Social media in disease surveillance

The Chicago Department of Public Health uses Twitter to identify cases of foodborne disease outbreak that analysed tweets that referred to food poisoning in the area. Using an app called Smart Chicago, the local government aimed to identify hotels and food joints that could be operating under unhygienic conditions (thereby flouting norms) where patrons were falling prey to food borne diseases. These establishments were then inspected. The New York City Department of Health has tied up with Yelp (a company that offers restaurant reviews, similar to India's Zomato) to create a similar app to help detect food borne diseases.

In the context of the Delhi dengue, a similar app may have been able to point at potential sources where such mosquitos could be breeding. After all, most food joints and street food hawkers in India tend to store fresh water for their patron's consumption and this is breeding ground for the dengue mosquito.

To ensure real time detection of flu in the US (which is the most common ailment and the reason for student/employee absenteeism in most cases), the government is collaborating with external research groups to forecast seasonal flu outbreaks. The current domestic influenza surveillance system informs public health decision-making, but it lags behind real-time flu activity. The goal of the new infectious disease forecasting is to provide a more-timely and forward-looking tool that predicts rather than monitors flu activity so that health officials can be more proactive in their prevention and mitigation responses.

For example, if it were possible to predict when and where flu activity will peak, health officials, health care providers and other partners could plan in advance to optimize the timing of flu vaccination clinics and communications outreach efforts around vaccination, as well as distribution of flu antiviral medications.

In the Delhi dengue context, if hospitals and healthcare professionals had used digital/social media to indicate the number of dengue cases that was being treated every hour, the severity of the situation would have come to light much earlier. The government could have responded faster with measures such as fumigation, distribution of vaccines, and even undertaking preventive checks in vulnerable localities.

India's population is not slowing down any time soon and healthcare funding as a percentage of GDP continues to shrink. Under such circumstances, digital disease surveillance can provide a cost effective way to manage disease and improve health care outcomes. It can bring together various stakeholders like healthcare professionals (who on their own don't tend to use digital media for creating awareness on diseases), patients (who need authentic medical information online), and healthcare providers (like hospitals and clinics who can share disease information) to comprehensively tackle disease and its symptoms.

Blockchain has the potential to transform healthcare in india

Recently we came to know about an interesting incident at a corporate wellness camp. The health workers recording the vital statistics of the participants were making key mistakes in recording the observations. A good example was the height of one of the participants was recorded wrongly as 147 centimeters instead of 157. Immediately the participant became obese as per the record. Similarly, BP was recorded wrongly for another participant. Though both mistakes were eventually rectified, we were left wondering how many such errors happen in the healthcare ecosystem daily and what the consequences of these errors would have been.

Also in our opinion having historical medical data would have given some guidance to the health workers collecting data. For example, the height of an adult would not change. Similarly looking at the pattern of previous Blood Pressure readings would have given the health workers an indication of whether they would need to take that reading again. Collecting, managing and storing healthcare information is the key to maintaining quality and improving care outcomes.

The experience from other countries is not very different. US-based healthcare organizations have spent around $ 93 Billion over the last five years in just data sharing costs? Surprised? Healthcare data can be complex – in part due to the non-linear nature of diagnosis and treatment, and also due to differing healthcare standards across regions in the world. Additionally, data privacy and other related laws can make healthcare information difficult to access and share. So much so that in many countries, including India, a patient may not have complete access to his/her medical record!

Considering that the next paradigm shift in healthcare is expected to come from the adoption of digital technologies – whether for patient experience or improved efficiency of hospital tasks – it is important to address current challenges around data sharing and access, lest they become hurdles to progress. In that context, Blockchain could be a saviour for the industry.

Blockchain is a continuously growing list of records, called blocks, which are linked and secured using cryptography. Each block contains, typically, a link to a previous block, a timestamp and transaction data. Transactions have to be approved by all users of the Blockchain to be stored and modifying an older block of data is impossible. Only updating of future records is permissible making the system secure (relatively speaking) and therefore reliable. This also means an entire Blockchain can serve as a secure ledger that records transactions, negating the need for multiple disparate trails of information.

We believe Indian healthcare has most to gain from the adoption of Blockchain technology. For starters, Blockchain allows all types of data to be integrated into the chain. This means one can add not just doctor prescriptions and treatment records but also nutrition information, fitness data, and recordings from medical devices (such as for blood pressure and diabetes patients) by patients themselves. Over time the presence of such longitudinal patient data means caregivers can better interpret disease symptoms and prescribe effective treatment that is customized to work for the patient. Currently, doctors rely on data from treating different patients to prescribe medication. The chances of success for such medication are about 50%. In many cases, doctors wait for feedback from patients to change the medication. With the availability of longitudinal patient data, doctors would know in advance what treatments are more likely to suit a patient in line with his/her health history.

If implemented over a large scale, Blockchain could help significantly lower healthcare costs in India. In addition, it can give multiple parties selective access to patient records ensuring data is not compromised. A survey report by IBM outlines the following healthcare areas benefiting from Blockchain: clinical trial records, patient health records, regulatory compliance, medical device data integration, treatment records, billing and claims, asset management (for hospital assets such as beds/ equipment available), and contract management (for hospitals).

In India we are proposing a new model for sharing and accessing Healthcare records over Blockchain. We are calling it Healthchain. The idea came from Priyank Jani, a technologist, who has been working on this concept for a while.

Healthchain is decentralized, distributed and anonymous which brings security, transparency, accessibility, and speed in EHR. Healthchain stored EHR and the immutable ledger maintenance makes it the single source of truth. All the records are cryptographically secured and need the owner's permission for access. Same way, it's distributed and decentralized so as a patient you need not rely on a single entity. It allows different participants like doctors, hospitals, Labs, insurance companies, and research agencies to be part of the Consortium. The patient is a base and key player of this solution makes him the owner of his records. He can access his records instantly across the globe; he can share or give timely permission to other participants to access his medical records and/or history for medical use. In fact, by sharing personal health records a patient may get some discount from the insurance agency and also get a reward from a health researcher.

In short, Healthchain gives rights and freedom to patients with their EHR by the power of Blockchain.

Currently, there are a few pilots running on Blockchain in Healthcare. Interestingly Estonia is already one of the most advanced nations when it comes to Blockchain implementation and has already been using Blockchain to deliver citizen and government services. They are planning to enable healthcare records of all their citizens on Blockchain. In 2016 Estonia digitized all health records and this is a critical first step towards the success of a future Blockchain implementation. Currently, all citizens in Estonia already carry a card with a unique id, similar to the Aadhar card in India. It will be interesting to see the results once all health records in Estonia are Blockchain enabled.

While there are many promises on Blockchain the adoption has been slow, these are primary due to 3 factors.

Use Cases- While technologists have developed proof of concepts, not too many good business cases have been developed, due to which many organisations hesitate while investing in Blockchain

Lack of Standards from Government – In India, the government is a big participant when it comes to adoption of technology. While in certain cases like Machine Learning and Artificial Intelligence the government has brought out standards, there has been no such movement on Blockchain.

Talent- Even if the first two criteria are met, there is still a lack of Blockchain talent in the country. While Academia is keen to partner with Industry, no concrete steps have been taken for the same.

Beyond Crypto Currency- A lot of discussions don't seem to go beyond Crypto Currency as a use case for Blockchain and Crytpo makes everyone sensitive as in a way it challenges the monetary policies and authority of India, there are other use cases which are more important but are often overlooked.

Traditionally, healthcare has been a laggard when it comes to embracing new technologies. However, the interest and exploration of Blockchain among other industries – finance and pharmaceuticals – may fuel Blockchain adoption in the healthcare industry in the coming years. But there is a technology that has emerged as a firm favourite among healthcare organisations in India and that is Machine learning.

Machine Learning and Analytics in Healthcare

Of the many advantages of technology since the arrival of computers is the ease with which data can be analysed to predict probable challenges as well solutions across various industries. By observing the prevalent trend and drawing comparisons, data analysis has the ability to greatly improve efficiency and decision-making capacity, based on solid statistics and research.

However, when faced with large data sets that include various patterns and trends, traditional analysis procedures often become inadequate. This is why more and more industries are increasingly moving towards analytics, especially in the field of healthcare. The Philips Innovation Campus has been using analytics to create solutions that would solve the healthcare issues.

Set up in 1996 the Philips Innovation Campus has more than 2000 research engineers, doctors and other medical experts that are building the healthcare systems of tomorrow.

They are not the only ones. GE Healthcare has been working on frugal innovation including portable ultrasounds and baby warmers. Siemens Healthineers recently announced plans to invest big in the healthcare technology space in India.

In a country like India, where the population is huge, the resultant pressures are visible in the infrastructure and healthcare system. It is common knowledge that majority of the people in the country do not have health insurance and given the high cost of treatment, families are often forced into financial crisis. While there are several good hospitals and healthcare facilities available in the tier one cities, many of them multinational players, the scenario is quite different in the tier two and rural areas.

Both the affordability and the availability of medical care are within reach for most people in the major metros. In the urban and semi-urban areas though, one finds that private players are usually replaced by nursing homes and district hospitals with a noticeable drop in the number of doctors available. This however, does serve as a possible emerging market for healthcare systems.

Of course, in the rural areas, it is the NGOs and the government that are required to be more involved through community and primary health centres. When compared with other countries like U.S., Western Europe, Japan, China, Brazil, Korea, South Africa and Thailand, India lags far behind in terms of beds, physicians and nurses. Not to mention a looming shortage of qualified doctors.

According to surveys conducted, non-communicable diseases such as cancer, diabetes, obesity, respiratory diseases, cardiovascular diseases, obesity and so on were the leading cause of death in India in 2008. Despite the rise in CVDs, the country has only about 5000 cardiologists with 300 new doctors added per year, and experts estimate that we also need twice the number of radiologists.

The biggest healthcare challenge facing the country today is not only the acute shortage of doctors and beds but also the affordability of treatment in Tier two and three cities and the rural areas. In such a scenario where there exist various contrasts within the same country, big data analytics can go a long way in improving the quality of treatment across all regions while keeping in mind its cost.

Analytics is of immense help when the data is too large and complex, i.e., it is difficult to capture, curate, store, search, share, transfer and analyse. By including descriptive, diagnostic, operational, predictive and prescriptive analytical values, big data analysis can be used fruitfully to mitigate future risks and plan the road ahead. Based on the information, healthcare facilities in India can be addressed better. The management of resources where there is a concern investment in suitable medical infrastructure and the workflow in hospitals can all be improved to a great degree.

Combined with programs like Disease Surveillance this can create the right input for citizens to take charge of your own health.

Machine Learning and Analytics are certainly the two pivots around which Healthcare would be delivered in the future, Things are going to be no different in India.

On the other hand, I think the use of these advanced technologies are the only way out to secure access to care of the billion plus in the country. All this is possible because of the confluence of machine learning and big data. Like I described in the previous chapter, weather satellites store tonnes of information and this is used courtesy Big Data to improve health parameters. Through machine learning these sites are able to provide contextual information to users. Healthcare can greatly benefit from these technologies and the good news is that they are already available in India.

Lybrate, is an online doctor consultation platform that enables users to communicate with doctors from anywhere, anytime. It is also one of the largest telemedicine platforms in India. The company has used technology to bridge the gap between patients and doctors by enabling them to talk with each other, thus democratizing healthcare in the country.

The huge data the company has generated, since it launched its platform in January 2015, made it introduce machine learning to suggest customized healthcare solutions to its users. Machine learning facilitates learning of users' interest and preferences over time to create a customized Health Feed, consisting of health tips from doctors and free answers by doctors to questions asked on the platform. This prevents users from getting bogged down by information not much of their interest.

Besides, when users ask queries on the platform, they do not know which doctor is best suited for them. Machine learning fixes this issue by deciphering users' query across more than 15 parameters in real time and help them get answers from relevant doctors.

So clearly Machine Learning and analytics are already being used by the government, industry and start-ups to improve standards of care. But there is lot left to be done, mainstream adoption is still far away with most hospitals and care providers still trying out these advanced technologies before the mainstream integration into the industry. A lot would depend on medical colleges and schools as well as they prepare to educate doctors and physicians.

Surprisingly the government is doing its bit to adopt technology.

SECTION 3

Healthcare initiatives by the Government

Ayushman Bharat

2018 saw the launch of the Ayushman Bharat Yojana by Prime Minister Shri Narendra Modi. It is a bold and ambitious step in the history of healthcare reforms in the nation. For the first time, a government has gone beyond lip sympathy on such a large scale.

The Ayushman Bharat Yojana is built on the sustainable development goals as defined by the United Nations and the objective is to leave no person behind in the field of healthcare. In other words, this scheme is in the spirit of universal healthcare and envisages to provide care, medicines, and diagnostics to all citizens, urban or rural, who are below the poverty line as described in the socio-economic census of India.

This scheme would be delivered on two key pillars

1. Health and Wellness Centers- to provide key diagnostics and free medicines

2. National Health Protection Scheme- Enabling cashless treatment for up to Rs 5 Lakhs for a family at a private (Empaneled) or Public Hospital. This like a federated model, and would depend on building a state health agency.

Some other key elements of the scheme

- Insurance benefit covers up to INR 5 lakhs per year per family

- The yearly premium for the insurance will be shared between the Central and State/UT government on a specified ratio

- State Health Agency(SHA) will be established at the state level for rolling out of the scheme.

- More than 100 million families can get benefit from the scheme (which covers about more than 40% of India's population).

- To make NHPS paperless and to encourage cashless transactions, the Ministry of Health and Family Welfare has partnered with NITI Aayog.

So how can you get involved?

Well if you are reading this then, you are most probably not eligible for the scheme. But it may be important for you to understand that almost 6-7 crore people fall below the poverty line every year because of medical expenses. So clearly there is a clear and urgent need to fix these. Most of the major schemes run by this government has been to fix the social infrastructure. The Swaach Bharat Campaign was laying the foundation of the health situation. Sanitation is the key reason why we got control over infectious diseases.

Here is what you can do-

1. I would encourage all of you to talk to your domestic helps, make them aware of the program.

2. Encourage them to register for the program

3. Read further on the scheme on the National Health Portal.

Let's see what else is the government doing in healthcare?

How the Government can drive technology adoption in healthcare?

The Indian government has been on the forefront of adopting technology for healthcare. The entire Ayushman Bharat scheme that we discussed earlier, is a cashless scheme running in the country, where more than 50 crore people have the access to hospitalisation where the bill is being paid by the government. In addition, applications like Aarogya Setu have enabled us to combat Covid19. A National Digital Health Mission has been launched with emphasis on access to care, digitization of health records in addition to privacy and security. Also, the government has released standards for areas like analytics and machine learning.

The government today is probably the largest provider of health care in India. Not only in the primary sector where the government provides almost 90% of all health care, but also in the secondary and the tertiary sector, the government still contributes about 50% of the number of doctors and beds in the country. I think the government has done a great job, especially the new government, which has come into power since 2014 has taken some significant steps in enhancing the image of healthcare in India.

What they have started with, is foundation elements like introducing standards for artificial intelligence standards for digital health and standards for the health stack, which are being adopted across the Indian healthcare ecosystem, and also being absorbed by many of the private entities in order to build scale into the healthcare ecosystem in

India. One of the challenges in India has been the lack of digitization and adoption of technology in healthcare, which has also led to serious issues like interoperability and scale of certain systems. For example, the electronic medical record system that can help patients, and or, and individuals to maintain the record across organizations or hospitals and refer the hospitals that they wish to with the launching of the standards, a lot of that would be taken care of as by following the India health stack. Many of these organizations would be able to, you know, board. The staff report the records of the, of the patient across the various entities. This would also be in the long term, with the establishment of an Electronic Health Record system country.

In the past, the government has led very ambitious schemes, like the one rate scheme for ambulance, by which by dialling the standard 108 number we can have an ambulance at your doorstep in record time. Similarly, the government also introduced the one or four number, which serves as a helpline and helpline for not only for your public health concerns but also for conditions like mental health and mental wellness, as well as, as recently been used as a forward headline across the country.

There have been certain controversies with the government as well. One of them being the use of the contact tracing apps that is being used for COVID-19 which primarily stems from the fact that we did not have the standards, or the approach in place for doing this in the beginning. But come, the end of the year, we won't have the standards from the India Health Stack in place and that should accelerate the growth and development of technologies, especially on the electronic health record side, and the electronic medical record side in the country.

One cannot forget the ambitious schemes that the Government has launched in the past, including the ESIC health care scheme which remains one of the largest health care schemes in the country catering to people that in the lower economic background. The comment also launched, the Ayushman Bharat scheme, which has helped in cashless transactions for up to 5 individuals per family below the poverty line for admissions for any number of conditions, the limit for the scheme is set at five lakhs as we are aware, and it can be availed on every year on here up to the five lakh limit.

The government needs to continue the push, when it comes to public health, and many of the schemes that are described in the past, especially areas like smoking cessation, or disease surveillance and population health, need to be taken nationally in order to provide us more insight on how to manage our health, while this is happening one scale, we need to continue to monitor the health ourselves and that is my hope and believe that after reading my words, and, and absorbing the philosophy that I've been following for a while, that most of you would be able to take care of your health.

In the meantime, let's also look at some of the schemes that the government has launched in the past.

As part of the Digital India initiative, the Prime Minister, Shri Narendar Modi has also launched the e-hospital program. The program enables patients to take appointments online and links premier institutes like AIIMS and NIMHANS. The other unique feature of this initiative is DigiLocker that enables patients to store sensitive information.

The system runs on the Online Registration System (ORS) which is a framework to link various hospitals across the country for Aadhaar based online registration and appointment system. In this scheme counter based OPD registration and appointment system through Hospital Management Information System (HMIS) has been digitalized. The application has been hosted on the cloud services of National Informatics Centre (NIC). The portal facilitates online appointments with various departments of different hospitals using eKYC data of Aadhaar number, if patient's mobile number is registered with UIDAI. And in case mobile number is not registered with UIDAI, it uses the patient's name. New patients will get appointment as well as Unique Health Identification (UHID) number.

But what took the cake was this low cost/ low tech solution from the Gujrat Government called E Mamta.

What does a successful eHealth initiative require?

Sophisticated Technology, armies of technical experts and senior doctors all working in tandem right? No wrong, if you follow the example set by the Gujrat government- all it needs is a mobile phone and a trained health worker.

The e-Mamta program run by the gujrat government has achieved good results with a technology as simple as the SMS.

In 2010 the infant mortality rate in Gujarat was 48 per 1000 live births. In a bid to improve these numbers and reduce the infant mortality rate the Gujarat government hit upon an idea to implement a mobile phone based program.

Under this program a health worker trained by the National Rural Health Mission (NRHM) travelled the length and breadth of Gujarat collecting information on expectant mothers and infants. This information was then sent back to the State Rural Health Mission (SRHM)) via SMS. The SMS was in Gujrati but typed in English letters. The information collected was very basic like the Pregnancy term, the immunizations taken and some other very basic vital statistics. The State rural health mission then collated this data and set up alerts for mothers and infants, who would be required to take vaccines or medicines as and when their pregnancy progressed.

These alerts were used to notify local health workers of the regions who reached out to these mothers to help them understand the plan and supply them with basic medication as required.

The plan worked and in 2012 the infant mortality rate dropped to 44 per 1000 live births. Now almost 480 Million families have registered for the e-Mamta program and are receiving the benefits of the program.

Seeing the success of the program many states like Andhra Pradesh and Uttrakhand are planning pilots and Nasscom had awarded the program with a social innovation award. Today e-Mamta covers 7 corporations, 172 Nagarpalikas and all villages in Gujrat.

So the bottom line is that countries like India can think in a frugally innovative fashion to provide healthcare and do not necessarily need huge investments in Infrastructure and technology. Hopefully E Mamta would be replicated in others parts of the country as well, as Gujarat shows the way even here. But let's learn more about the primary healthcare system in India, and our frontline health workers, ASHA and Anganwadi volunteers.

Strengthening the primary healthcare system

One thing that COVID has exposed is the gross unpreparedness of the Indian healthcare system to deal with pandemics. But it also exposed how little we knew about the situation on the ground. Data available is inadequate and most of the data especially from the villages and districts is not captured.

At the front line for the fight against disease and other illnesses is the Indian Primary Care system. This system is mostly run by ASHA (Accredited Social Health Activists) and While they have been around since the recommendations of the Bhore Committee in 1943, it is easy to see how they are ill-prepared to deal with spread of disease.

Below is some data that I have been able to ascertain from public sources.

Number of ASHA Workers	9,00,000
Number of primary health centers	25,000
Average Salaries of ASHA Workers	INR 2,000/PM
Average costs incurred by ASHA Workers	INR 800/PM

So this is the on-ground scenario. These workers have to fill multiple forms for child care, maternal care among others, and then they make 10-15 home visits per day. There are key reasons why ASHA workers are important.

1.   They are local to an area, they understand the local customs and traditions

2.   They have the trust of the community (communities in rural India do not like to discuss their health with strangers)

3.   While they are part timers, going from home to home makes them the best eyes and ears for the healthcare system

But given their situation and low pay, would it be interesting to see what we can do to help their situation. The government is spending close to INR 5000 Crore on the Ayushman Bharat Program. Next year the outlay is close to 10,000 Crore. But at a fraction of this cost, we can increase the pay for the ASHA workers and get much better coverage to prevent patients from getting hospitalized. But can Healthcare become an election issue? Post Covid 19? Well the answer is not that simple. Let's find out.

Why are politicians not interested in healthcare?

Earlier in the book I had discussed what Dr. Devi Shetty had said about politics and healthcare. He felt healthcare would become a poll issue after Covid 19. But in my opinion it would be very difficult, this might be controversial but well we have nearly come to the end of the book and there is always a little room for controversy.

Given the historically low percentage of budget allocated to public health in India, can Covid19 realistically push the government to prioritise this area?

An analysis of select 2014 election manifestos indicates that we may be woefully behind on the path to a more comprehensive health plan for citizens.

- India spends about 1.2% of its GDP on health services and in 2018 this number went up to 1.4%. However, this is still significantly lower than the time and efforts allocated to areas like physical infrastructure development and jobs.

- Women Led parties had more space dedicated to healthcare in their election manifestos (AIADMK – 6% and TMC – 5%). AAP follows closely with 4%, whereas national parties BJP and Indian National Congress (INC) dedicated around 2.3% and 2.1%, respectively. Interestingly, the AIADMK appears to have implemented many of its promises, given that Tamilnadu leads on several health parameters, the TMC in West Bengal needs a stronger implementation policy to suitably action on its promise.

- Most parties tend to pay little attention to preventive health. There is almost no mention of areas like nutrition in election manifestos and while the BJP manifesto does talk about Swachh Bharat, there is no mention of ways to tie that back to measuring health outcomes. The INC manifesto talks about malnutrition and mentions Anaemia and HIV but does not spell out anything concrete in terms of action plans to prevent or tackle the disease.

- All election manifestos considered for analysis missed addressing non-communicable diseases and the measures to tackle them. Given the high incidence of non-communicable diseases such as diabetes and hypertension in India, this is a glaring miss.

- Most of the focus on health in manifestos is on building hospitals – more beds and more clinics and so on. But there is no focus on the quality of care provided at these centres or the variety of ailments they can treat. One cannot provide hospitalisation and expect improvement in the state of health without tackling the underlying social and sanitation causes for the ailments.

- Strangely, while the focus remains on building new facilities, there is no mention of improving existing primary health centres and community health centres that have suffered from decades of neglect. Even in Ayushman Bharat these have not been addressed. While the insurance part of Ayushman Bharat is doing well, the wellness program can be significantly improved.

- There is no mention of disease surveillance in any manifesto. This is surprising considering most developing countries in the world have some semblance of proactive disease surveillance to curb the spread of disease and manage its citizens' health.

In summary, even if all that has been promised in the election manifesto is delivered, it would not make a dent in the state of health in the country.

Why is this so?

Historically India missed the boat in prioritising healthcare reforms recommended by the Bhore committee in 1946 particularly the delivery of health at the grass root levels through primary health centres (PHCs).

Further, religious beliefs that tie poor health to karma and a generally fatalistic outlook have ensured hospitals and external care providers are seen as the last resort for patients. Preventive healthcare was largely provided at home. In line with this, the government has not undertaken research connecting the health of its citizens to their productivity. For instance, a study in the UK found that those who smoked were twice as likely to take time off work. Another study found that workers with obesity (BMI over 30) annually took an average of three sick days more than those with normal weight (BMI less than 25), and those with severe obesity (BMI over 35) took six days more. In India, a large population and limited availability of jobs means employment remains a bigger issue than health for the government.

The relatively affordable cost of healthcare so far has also meant citizens have remained negligent about lifestyle diseases. Until recently health insurance wasn't understood and perhaps without the tax exemption many citizens may not opt for it.

Until the time healthcare is viewed as a discretionary spend, political parties may see no value in contesting elections on the plank of better healthcare for citizens. Citizens themselves need to demand for better health from its government for parties to take the issue seriously. A possible reason why some of the Southern states have overall better health indicators is the relatively high proportion of senior citizen population that resides alone, without support from younger people who tend to live outside the state/ country. This changing demographic of voters may have prompted political parties in the region to place greater emphasis on public health and deliver results.

In addition, states like Karnataka and Kerala have prospered from the investments from the princely states. Tamilnadu alone benefitted by keeping public health distinct from Health Services, this is one of the few states that implemented this recommendation from the Bhore Committee recommendations. So unfortunately for you the onus is back on you. Unless you as an individual demand better healthcare politicians would not like to improve the state of care in the country.

All's well that ends well

Congratulations on finishing the book. I think you've taken the first major step towards owing your health. Like I said in the beginning, health is an important factor. It's the key to happiness. And it's very important that you take charge of it.

The reality is that if you don't take charge of it, nobody else will. Nobody else can. The reasons for that are many folds.

Nobody knows you better than you.

Nobody can motivate you better than you.

And finally, nobody can take charge of you and your health as well as you can

While you've gone through this book, I would also recommend that you spread this message, talk to others, and ask them to take charge of their health and follow the principles that are described in the book.

Essentially, first, Own two twin killers of the modern knowledge worker of the white-collar worker. That is diabetes and hypertension. Keep track of your sugar levels. Keep track of your blood pressure. I think prevention is the key here. Make sure that you indulge in practices that help you reduce stress. Stress and these two conditions are co-related. Follow very basic techniques to keep these under control. I think that is another area where the brain tries to fool us to make us believe that, we've eaten adequately, but in reality, we may have not eaten at all. Again you know there are nutrition apps available I personally use HealthifyMe but you can use any app that you fancy or you have to go to the Android App Store or the or the Apple Store and find an app which has a good rating and especially if it's an Android app. Make sure its security features are well vetted.

Number two, look at detecting a lot of the deficiencies that affect us. The three common ones, in my opinion, are vitamin D, Vitamin B 12 and Thyroid. If you take care of these three, you are gold. Mostly foundationally, your health will remain fine. The second layer, which I encourage you to take care of is your physical fitness. Again, I do not recommend for you to go all Rambo, in running around looking for gyms, getting yourself into physical injuries by pushing yourself across the limit.

What I'm talking about is basic tenets like walking, cycling, swimming, anything that you can incorporate in your life. Make sure that you're at least spending about 150 minutes a week in outdoor physical exercise that is useful not only for your health but also helps with your Vitamin D Levels. And the most important thing, like in measuring and detecting is ensuring that you keep a record of your activity, see the brain has a very interesting way of fooling us, and making us feel that we have had adequate exercise, while we may have missed exercise for a long time. So, keep track of your workouts, keep track of the minutes you spend use basic tools, all these tools are available to you on your phone, or use Google Fit. You can use that as well.

Then comes our interesting feature on mental wellness, where it is important for you to keep a healthy mind. Here I've collaborated extensively with Dr. Kiran, who himself is a psychiatrist, from the NIMHANs in Bangalore and Dr. Ashwin Naik founder of Mana Wellness. And we've talked about a lot of things that you can do, including meditation, yoga, physical fitness regular consultation with your counsellor with your doctors.

You are, what your mind tells you. If your mind tells you are well, you're well if your mind tells you you're sick you're sick. So, it's very important for you to keep your mind healthy and act, follow very active lifestyles.

A big section on habits. Where do I begin, you know, usually when you talk about habits we talk about tobacco smoking and alcohol consumption. But you know what I what I realized, personally, is we have to add two more elements to it, and which are sugar and salt. Sugar is a very addictive substance and sugar is now present in almost every processed food we see around us.

Even harmless items like soup, have a lot of sugar because sugar not only enhances taste, but it's also a great preservative. Watch out for sugar monitor your sugar levels as well make out of the habit of having too much added sugar in your diet. It's very difficult to eliminate it tried to reduce it step by step and bring it to an optimal level, there are guidelines on how much sugar is required for a man and a woman living a sedentary lifestyle, and we should keep ourselves below it. I would, however, put no limits on natural sugar sugars that occur in fruits or vegetables. I think those are fine they don't hurt us as much as anger toward us.

Similarly, the other habit that has crept up on us is salt intake, again you know processed food is a big beneficiary of increased amounts of salt because salt is also good preservative, and salt makes you very dehydrated, which, which makes you want to consume water. And that leads to water retention and this invariably leads to weight gain. So, in habits, though I talked about alcohol quite a lot, and I talk about smoking. I do talk a lot about salt and sugar, because I think these are two. Usual Suspects very readily available part of every house but are very dangerous and very habit for me.

The last point I want to make on habits is smoking. You know I don't want to preach on the effects of smoking. If you are reading this you're smart you're intelligent, you must be working for a corporate setup and you must be having so many smoking cessation policies in your organization that I don't want to, you know, overindulge and preach on you. That's why I've taken a very counterintuitive approach, I've looked at the economics of smoking. And this is a deliberate ploy on my part to talk to you about how you're contributing to the growth of Indian economy through smoking. And it does, it's, it's doing a lot of harm to you. At the same time, adding no nutritional value. So I've taken a simple example of the cost. The average costs of smoking, which amounts to almost 1200 rupees, a month. And I think the best thing you can do is keep that money in your pocket. Keep that figure in your mind and add it to your bank balance and do wonderful things with it, rather than indulging in something that adds no nutritional value, and in turn would cause greater harm and financial harm at a later stage in terms of first hospitalization, then in the end I talk about two important aspects, your lifestyle and your genetics.

In lifestyle, I discuss areas like flexible working timings, I discuss important areas that should be addressed, like sleep, yoga, meditation, ayurveda, which I believe are more of lifestyle changes that you can make for prolonging functional and fruitful life on genetics. There is not much you can do as these are the genes you have inherited, obviously, but you can also even learn more about what are the disease conditions you're predisposed to. And then finally, what the government has been doing for us. A bit of controversy on the government side but hey what is life and what is a book without, without some controversy.

I would thank you once again for taking this choice when making this choice, reading a book that will help you change your life forever. This is the only body you came in with and it's probably the only body with which you will leave, with the way things stand. Please take care of yourself. Stay healthy. Stay happy and looking forward to a very fruitful and healthy life ahead.

Own Your Health, remember no one else can do…

(Ends)

Sources

https://www.ncbi.nlm.nih.gov/pmc/articles/PMC4933534/

https://healthcare-in-india.net/medical-education/the-problem-of-diabetes-in-india-and-how-to-control-it-a-detailed-analysis/

https://www.diabetes.co.uk/what-is-hba1c.html

https://healthcare-in-india.net/medical-education/the-problem-of-diabetes-in-india-and-how-to-control-it-a-detailed-analysis/

https://healthcare-in-india.net/public-health-2/how-alcoholism-is-creating-a-socio-economic-problem-in-india/

https://www.ncbi.nlm.nih.gov/pmc/articles/PMC5648391/

https://www.thehindubusinessline.com/news/science/smoking-causes-over-11-deaths-india-among-top-4-countries-report/article9618981.ece#

https://www.indianmirror.com/indian-industries/tobacco.html

https://en.wikipedia.org/wiki/Smoking_in_India#cite_note-8

https://healthcare-in-india.net/healthcare-delivery/why-hypertension-the-silent-killer-and-how-you-can-control-your-blood-pressure/

https://healthcare-in-india.net/public-health-2/post-covid19-will-healthcare-become-a-poll-issue-in-india/

https://healthcare-in-india.net/healthcare-technology/indian-healthcare-wearable-fitness-tracker-market-set-to-explode/

https://healthcare-in-india.net/healthcare-technology/indian-healthcare-wearable-fitness-tracker-market-set-to-explode/

https://healthcare-in-india.net/healthcare-delivery/malnutrition-and-not-obesity-is-indias-biggest-health-challenge-for-the-21ˢᵗ-century/

https://healthcare-in-india.net/wellness/why-it-is-important-for-children-in-india-to-catch-up-on-lost-growth/

https://healthcare-in-india.net/public-health-2/right-nutrition-is-the-key-to-the-health-of-senior-citizens-in-india/

https://healthcare-in-india.net/public-health-2/malnutrition-in-india-one-problem-many-solutions/

https://www.ncbi.nlm.nih.gov/pmc/articles/PMC4317993/

https://healthcare-in-india.net/public-health-2/right-nutrition-is-the-key-to-the-health-of-senior-citizens-in-india/

https://healthcare-in-india.net/healthcare-technology/nutrition-first-how-an-app-seeks-to-make-people-aware-of-their-food-habits/

https://www.health.harvard.edu/blog/vitamin-d-whats-right-level-2016121910893

https://healthcare-in-india.net/healthcare-delivery/how-vitamin-d-deficiency-could-be-silently-killing-you/

https://timesofindia.indiatimes.com/city/ahmedabad/That-bowl-of-cereals-may-not-be-healthy/articleshow/3995166.cms

https://healthcare-in-india.net/public-health-2/is-cornflakes-for-breakfast-a-healthy-proposition-for-india/

https://youtu.be/ywbXI9ARe2U

https://healthcare-in-india.net/public-health-2/is-cornflakes-for-breakfast-a-healthy-proposition-for-india/

https://pdfs.semanticscholar.org/44f4/da7f3149197c992f0de33e036e6ea6b078f9.pdf

https://en.wikipedia.org/wiki/Idli#cite_note-12

https://www.thehindubusinessline.com/news/national/amma-canteens-in-chennai-to-serve-food-for-free-till-lockdown-ends/article31416858.ece#

https://healthcare-in-india.net/wellness/how-the-humble-idli-can-solve-the-nutrition-problem-in-india/

https://www.thenewsminute.com/article/how-digital-disease-surveillance-systems-could-have-prevented-delhi-dengue-outbreak-50556

https://www.ncbi.nlm.nih.gov/pmc/articles/PMC1120878/

https://www.philips.co.in/a-w/about-philips/philips-innovation-center/about-us.html

https://healthcare-in-india.net/wellness/how-big-data-can-help-healthcare/

https://healthcare-in-india.net/healthcare-technology/machine-learning-and-big-data-for-improved-healthcare-in-india/

https://healthcare-in-india.net/healthcare-technology/is-indian-healthcare-ready-for-big-data-and-analytics/

http://e-mamta.gujarat.gov.in/

https://healthcare-in-india.net/healthcare-technology/e-mamta-a-great-example-of-low-cost-ehealth-initiative-from-gujrat-government/

https://healthcare-in-india.net/wellness/the-curious-rise-of-mental-illness-in-india/

https://www.rediff.com/news/report/rediff-labs-how-india-consumes-tobacco-part-2/20180802.htm

https://health.ri.gov/healthrisks/salt/#:~:text=Too%20much%20
salt%20increases%20the,%2C%20heart%20disease%2C%20and%20
stroke.

https://healthcare-in-india.net/healthcare-delivery/3-health-benefits-
of-practicing-yoga/

https://healthcare-in-india.net/public-health-2/post-covid19-will-
healthcare-become-a-poll-issue-in-india/

https://healthcare-in-india.net/wp-content/uploads/2020/07/
Healthcare-and-Democracy_Can-Healthcare-become-an-election-
issues-in-India.pdf

https://healthcare-in-india.net/wp-content/uploads/2020/08/Patient-
Experience-in-India.pdf

https://healthcare-in-india.net/healthcare-delivery/genetic-risk-score-
to-provide-early-detection-of-heart-disease/

https://healthcare-in-india.net/life-sciences/genetics-and-scientific-
research-into-the-management-of-dengue-in-india/

https://healthcare-in-india.net/healthcare-technology/new-guidelines-
launched-for-telemedicine-practice-by-medical-council-of-india-and-
niti-aayog/

https://healthcare-in-india.net/healthcare-technology/new-guidelines-
launched-for-telemedicine-practice-by-medical-council-of-india-and-
niti-aayog/

https://fit.thequint.com/health-news/technology-making-headway-in-
healthcare-2

https://healthcare-in-india.net/mental-health/managing-your-mental-
health-and-wellness-during-covid-19/

https://www.ncbi.nlm.nih.gov/pmc/articles/
PMC4449495/#:~:text=Serotonin%20is%20a%20

neurotransmitter%20that,serotonin%20available%20to%20brain%20
cells.

https://news.harvard.edu/gazette/story/2017/04/over-nearly-80-
years-harvard-study-has-been-showing-how-to-live-a-healthy-and-
happy-life/

About the Author

Dr. Vikram Venkateswaran is a doctor who switched over to technology based healthcare management systems, and believes in taking charge of one's health. He has worked with major healthcare systems in the US, India and the UK. To effect a change in how healthcare is perceived and delivered in India, he started Healthcare India, a digital platform to focus on personal health management, public health, technology and care delivery in India. Started in 2010, Healthcare India is among the top 100 global platforms on Healthcare Technology.

He studied at DPS PK Puram, New Delhi, and then attended the Manipal College of Dental Surgery (MCODS). After running a dental practice in Delhi for 6 years, he completed an MBA from IMT Ghaziabad, specialising in Marketing and Strategy. In 2013 he was awarded the Distinguished Toastmasters award by Toastmasters International. Dr. Vikram lives in Bangalore, India, with his wife and two children. He can be reached at drvikram@healthcare-in-india.net

Reviews

Own it.

Owning your health is probably the most important activity that you should indulge in. Dr. Vikram captures the essence of health and the role technology plays in the same

Ankit Rajiv Jindal
Founder - Friends for Inclusion

Health is the most foundational layer of life. The rest of the layers like wealth, social life, professional life are all built on top of this foundation and they have no real meaning in the absence of physical and mental health. If you don't own your health, what can you truly own?

Dr. Sudhakar Varanasi
Healthcare Mentor and Innovator

A must read

Health tech is an essential catalyst in providing safe, affordable and timely healthcare which is critical to the outcome of our rapidly growing nation. *Own your health* sets the stage for how citizens can adapt to the future health ecosystem.

Dr. Sumeet Kad
Cluster Head - Enterprise States
Roche Products (India) Pvt. Ltd.

One of the biggest casualties of the modern digitized living are our eyes. Own Your Health discusses simple ways to care for your eyes.

Dr. Abhiyan Kumar Pattnaik
Director Dr. Pattnaik's Laser Eye Clinic